T0313947

The Way of Medicine

NOTRE DAME STUDIES IN MEDICAL ETHICS
AND BIOETHICS

O. Carter Snead, series editor

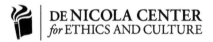

The purpose of the Notre Dame Studies in Medical Ethics and Bioethics series, sponsored by the de Nicola Center for Ethics and Culture, is to publish works that explore the ethical, cultural, and public questions arising from advances in biomedical technology, the practice of medicine, and the biosciences.

The Way of Medicine

Ethics and the Healing Profession

FARR CURLIN

and

CHRISTOPHER TOLLEFSEN

University of Notre Dame Press
Notre Dame, Indiana

Library of Congress Control Number: 2021942665

ISBN: 978-0-268-20085-5 (Hardback)
ISBN: 978-0-268-20086-2 (Paperback)
ISBN: 978-0-268-20084-8 (WebPDF)
ISBN: 978-0-268-20087-9 (Epub)

To our spouses, Kimberly Curlin and Laurie Tollefsen,
who merit more thanks and praise
than we can possibly give here

CONTENTS

A Perplexed Physician

I sensed early in my medical training that something had gone wrong at the heart of our profession. I came to medical training confident that caring for those who are sick would readily fit into my vocation as a Christian, not because Christians have a lock on healing—by no means. Rather, because everyone—whether Jew, Christian, Muslim, atheist, or other—knows that healing is good work, even "God's work." I knew that modern physicians had gotten involved in a few practices—elective abortion and assisted suicide in particular—opposed both by traditional Christianity and by traditional medical ethics. But these practices were on the margins, I thought, exceptions to medicine's otherwise consistent orientation toward healing. It did not take long for me to realize that I was mistaken—that these overtly controversial practices expressed deeper changes at the heart of the medical profession. Having come over the second half of the twentieth century to "provide" all kinds of interventions that were not so obviously a part of healing those who are sick, physicians could no longer say what it meant to heal. In seven years of medical school and residency training, I do not recall a medical educator ever encouraging me or my fellow trainees to consider what medicine is *for*.

How could we clinicians-in-training find our way if our teachers could not tell us where that way leads? We learned to take our bearings by setting aside the question of what medicine is for and instead focusing on getting where we were asked to go as efficiently and effectively as possible. Those were the heady days of evidence-based medicine.

Medical educators advocated "the conscientious, explicit, and judicious use of current best evidence in making decisions about the care of individual patients."[1] Unfortunately, our teachers had much less to say about what norms we should conscientiously uphold and by what standards we should evaluate whether our use of evidence had been judicious. The resulting vacuum was filled with the default norm of contemporary medicine: support the autonomous choices of patients as long as doing so is not illegal, infeasible, or unequivocally harmful.

Indeed, the language of conscience and judgment proved to be the residue of a tradition of practice that the profession of medicine seemed determined to leave behind—a tradition associated with paternalism, patriarchy, and other specters of a repressive past. To avoid recapitulating the injustices of that past, we learned to ask not what ought to be done but *who decides* what ought to be done. After all, what would give a physician the authority to judge what is good for someone else? Shouldn't patients decide what happens to their bodies? We were taught various ethical principles we might invoke to describe a clinical decision, but we also learned that in the end only the patient could decide which of these principles should govern in their particular case. Being "patient-centered," we discovered, meant respecting patients' right to judge what is good for them. So we made patient preferences our guide, and we resisted the temptation to impose our own values under the pretense of conscience and clinical judgment. The safest route was to separate the personal from the professional, keeping the former from intruding on the latter.

I have never made peace with this notion of separating the personal from the professional. I had set out to practice medicine because caring for the sick seemed to fit into the Christian vocation to love God and one's neighbor. In training, however, Christian commitments largely were construed as "personal values" that must be kept from interfering with my professional obligations. While I puzzled over how that could be so, I observed that separating the personal from the professional reified the sterility and detachment of clinical encounters that left patients dissatisfied and physicians dispirited.

How did we end up with this idea that medicine requires compartmentalizing the personal away from the professional? How did medical educators end up teaching that good physicians must be willing to be bad Christians, Jews, or Muslims?

I did not find satisfying answers to these questions, but who was I to challenge the status quo? This ancient profession went on before me and will go on after me, whether I like it or not. Perhaps in time I would see that by keeping my personal and professional lives separate, focusing on scientific data, and deferring to others to tell me what to pursue, I would become a better physician than I had imagined. I would find that to love my neighbors means to do what they ask me to do even when that goes against my better judgment. And if I could not reconcile my personal moral sensibilities with the standards of the profession, I could find a different line of work. I had not been conscripted, after all.

But further experience only confirmed my misgivings that the medical profession had lost its way. Indeed, in the name of respect for patient autonomy, the profession seemed to have given up any claim to know where that way should lead. The medical profession trains its members to defer to patients regarding what goals physicians are to pursue, reserving to the clinician the authority only to insist that those ends be pursued in a scientifically informed and effective manner. So, for example, a physician cannot know whether he should sterilize a patient or offer her assisted reproductive technologies until and unless the patient tells him what she wants. The physician can decide, however, which surgical technique is most effective for sterilization and which exogenous hormones will effectively hyperstimulate the ovaries. Many medical ethicists likewise have abandoned any claim to know what medicine is for. As a member of the clinical ethics faculty at a premier academic medical center, I joined colleagues in spirited debates about who was authorized to make a particular clinical decision, but we almost never discussed what that person should decide, or why. We had learned to police ourselves to avoid the presumption of claiming to know what good medicine required for this or that patient.

Meanwhile, in the hospital I watched countless physicians bend over backward to give patients and their family members all the options for their cases and to avoid "imposing" any judgment regarding what was best for the patients. Physicians routinely would tell family members of critically ill patients that the decision to continue or discontinue life-sustaining technology was not the physicians' to make, or even the family's to make. Rather, all were obligated to set aside their judgment about what would be good for the patient and instead choose what the patient would choose if the patient could choose for himself. When families did not choose as the physicians hoped they would, the physicians would retreat to their workrooms to grumble about unrealistic family members who were in denial. Doctors resent continuing unreasonable efforts to keep patients alive, but they do not see any other option. They have internalized the axiom that only patients, or their surrogates, can say what is good for them.

The same demoralized ethos carried over into the outpatient setting, where, for example, physicians were long taught that the patient's pain was what the patient said it was, and the physician was obligated to treat that pain until the patient said it was relieved. Those of us who practice hospice and palliative medicine have been taught that relieving pain and other symptoms is not enough; we are also to maximize quality of life and to minimize suffering. No one but the patient can say whether we have achieved that goal, so we must follow patients' preferences closely, including their preferences regarding how and when to die.

Physicians have become particularly reticent to say what medicine is for in the domain of sexuality and reproduction. A patient once asked me to prescribe Viagra because he was having difficulty sustaining an erection when having sex with his wife, though he had no such problems when with his mistress. My colleagues were ambivalent as to how I should respond. On one hand, it seemed strange to facilitate this man's infidelity to his wife. On the other, the drug was safe, legal, and permitted by the profession; who was I to judge? A homosexual man whom I had treated for high blood pressure asked me to help him and his partner figure out how to get a baby through in vitro fertilization (IVF) using an anonymous egg donor and a gestational surrogate. My colleagues were agreed that I should accommodate his request, at least by referring the patient to the assisted reproductive technology clinic. For a few years, I took night calls for my university's student health service, and some nights more students called to ask for prescriptions for "emergency contraceptives" than called because they were sick. I found myself asking, "What does giving people all of these things they want have to do with practicing medicine?"

One might think that deferring to patients about the goals of medicine would lead to greater patient satisfaction, but that is not what I have observed. Instead, by relinquishing their professional authority, physicians seem to have given third parties a free hand to intrude on and govern the physicians' experiences and their patients', to the chagrin of both. Today, patients and clinicians alike are harried by impersonal forces along paths they hardly understand. Patients ask for whatever the latest pharmaceutical commercial, or the latest social fashion or anxiety, recommends. Meanwhile, doctors submit to the demands of Medicare and other insurers, bean counters tracking relative value units (RVUs), and, most of all, the electronic medical record. Practitioners may start by asking a patient, "How can I help you today?," but they soon turn their attention to the invisible social engineer standing in the corner of every exam room, armed with a checklist the doctor must follow in order to ensure that she provides quality care that is safe and "value-based." Neither patients nor physicians call the shots, and both feel helpless to change the system.

Helplessness leads both to demoralization and to detachment. Why would anyone want to practice medicine if doing so meant setting aside their religious aspirations, their ethical judgment, and their longing to connect with patients on a human level? Why would anyone aspire to serve as an efficient cog in a vast, bureaucratically structured healthcare industry? In this situation, physicians and other healthcare practitioners give up the quest to find—much less pursue—what medicine is *for*. The work to which medical practitioners thought they were called becomes a job to tolerate. Their patients present them not with the privilege of cooperating in pursuit of healing but with the burden of satisfying demands that clinicians frequently resent. Medical practitioners, then, need self-care and work-life balance to mitigate the threat of medicine to their integrity and their flourishing and to keep them from walking away from the practice of medicine altogether. That, at least, is how it has seemed to me.

If you are a physician and this account resonates at all with your own experience, this book is for you. Moreover, if you long to recover a way of practicing medicine that can truly be seen as a "calling," intrinsically rewarding work to which you can happily commit the best of your time, attention, and energy, then read on. We hope you will learn to better see and to say what you know, and so be equipped to continue the worthy adventure of practicing medicine.

THIS BOOK HAS been written by a practicing physician, Farr Curlin, and a philosophy professor, Christopher Tollefsen. It grew out of a seminar we have taught together for almost ten years, but it is inspired by what I have experienced and observed in my training and practice as a clinician and medical ethicist. Some readers may recognize in my account their own unease and uncertainty about what medicine has become.

Farr Curlin, MD

ACKNOWLEDGMENTS

This book originated in an annual week-long seminar in medical ethics that we have taught since 2011, initially sponsored by the Witherspoon Institute in Princeton, New Jersey, and now by the Arete Initiative at Duke University. We are indebted to those whose vision and leadership have made the seminar possible, especially Robby George and Luis Tellez, as well as those who have given hospitality to the scores of clinician trainees who have joined us over the years, including Patrick Hough, Felix Miller, Phil Braun, and John Rose. And we are indebted to our students in those seminars, who have committed their lives to the practice of medicine and whose sincere questions, contentions, and arguments made invaluable contributions to this book.

Medicine, as we argue here, is a *practice*, as is the doing and teaching of philosophy. We could never have gotten started in understanding either practice without the help of our teachers, among whom Farr notes particularly Drs. Carl Kraus, Mark Siegler, Daniel Sulmasy, and Leon Kass; Chris acknowledges with gratitude three philosophers who have died since our work on this book began: Joseph Boyle, Germain Grisez, and H. Tristram Engelhardt.

As this book has taken shape over the past several years, a number of colleagues have gifted us with their critiques of our arguments. We thank Jason Amaral, Ryan Anderson, Jeff Baker, Jeffrey Bishop, Chip Denton, Lydia Dugdale, H. Tristram Engelhardt, Nick Epley, Margaret Houck, Ana Iltis, Lauris Kaldjian, Daniel Kim, Scott Kim, Warren Kinghorn, Brett McCarty, Abraham Nussbaum, Brian Quaranta, Jon Tilburt, John Yoon, and anonymous reviewers of the University of

Notre Dame Press. None of these agree with us on every point, and some disagree with us on major points. The deficiencies of the book are our own, but these share credit for any of the book's merits, as do those who have helped us in the editing process, including Judith Heyhoe, Luke Olsen, and Bob Land.

Farr is particularly grateful to colleagues at the Trent Center for Bioethics, Humanities, and History of Medicine at Duke University and those in Duke Divinity School's Initiative on Theology, Medicine, and Culture (TMC). Both of these institutional spaces foster unusually fertile environments for inquiring about the moral and theological dimensions of the practice of medicine. Chris thanks the James Madison Program at Princeton University, the Eudaimonia Institute at Wake Forest University, and his own University of South Carolina. Each has been home to some of the drafting of this book, and colleagues and friends at each deserve much thanks.

We have written about many of the ideas in this book in other places. A number of the arguments and examples appear elsewhere, in particular the following, which are listed in the order in which they were published:

Farr Curlin, "Hospice and Palliative Medicine's Attempt at an Art of Dying," in Lydia S. Dudgale, ed., *Dying in the Twenty-First Century: Toward a New Ethical Framework for the Art of Dying Well* (Cambridge, MA: MIT Press, 2015), 47–66.

Y. Tony Yang and Farr A. Curlin, "Why Physicians Should Oppose Assisted Suicide," *Journal of the American Medical Association* 315, no. 3 (2016): 247–248.

Christopher Tollefsen, "Abortion," in Bob Fisher, *Ethics, Left and Right: The Moral Issues that Divide Us* (New York: Oxford University Press, 2020), 340–48.

Farr A. Curlin and Christopher O. Tollefsen, "Medicine against Suicide: Sustaining Solidarity with those Diminished by Illness and Debility," in *Christian Bioethics*, forthcoming.

Christopher Tollefsen and Farr Curlin, "Solidarity, Trust, and Christian Faith in the Doctor-Patient Relationship," *Christian Bioethics*, forthcoming.

In addition, an earlier version of chapter 10 was published as

Farr A. Curlin and Christopher O. Tollefsen, "Conscience and the Way of Medicine," *Perspectives in Biology and Medicine* 62, no. 3 (2019): 560–75, reprinted with permission.

Introduction

A Profession in Crisis

Medical practitioners and those who want to become such practitioners face basic questions: What is medicine? What is medicine *for*? What does it mean to be a good doctor? Their answers seem essential to the practice of medicine and to understanding its moral norms. The absence of answers to these questions—or incoherent or incorrect answers—would seem to prefigure a crisis for both medicine and medical ethics. For without correct and coherent answers, practitioners of medicine cannot properly orient themselves within their profession, nor even think of their practice as a profession at all. And without some account of what the medical profession *professes*—without an account of medicine's purpose or end—ethicists rely on norms that bear only contingent relationships to the activities of medical professionals. Ethicists fail, in other words, to articulate an *ethics of medicine* in the proper sense.

We believe that medicine, and hence medical ethics, is in precisely this sort of crisis. Medicine has lost its way because it lacks clarity about where the way should lead. We no longer have a shared public understanding of what medicine is for, of what the *end of medicine* is or should be. Rather, medicine has substituted for its once clearly recognized purpose something amorphous, subjective, and shadowy. As a consequence, the norms that medical professionals and professional ethicists bring to medical practice are devoid of objective content and radically deficient for guiding doctors and protecting patients.

1

THE PROVIDER OF SERVICES MODEL FOR MEDICINE

In answer to the question "What is medicine?," according to the *provider of services model*, medicine comprises a set of technical skills that are to be put to work to satisfy patient-client preferences. Healthcare workers are providers of services, and these services are undertaken for the sake of patient well-being, understood principally in terms of satisfying the patient's wishes.[1]

Every culture gets the medical practice it deserves, and in our culture medical practice is dominated by a consumerist understanding, where well-being is understood in terms of the patient's desires being satisfied. Efforts to identify an ethical framework capable of guiding practitioners and patients in our time have resulted in consequentialism, contractarianism, and, most prominently, principlism—the framework that gives us the familiar "four principles" of medical ethics.[2] In the context of an individualist and consumerist environment, however, these efforts all tend to default to three norms: what the law permits, what is technologically possible, and what the patient wants.

Thus, according to the provider of services model, if an intervention is permitted by law, is technologically possible, and is autonomously desired by the patient, medical practitioners should provide the intervention. Indeed, they may be professionally obligated to do so.[3] After all, these norms fit our expectations of other providers of services. The good folks who provide us with Wi-Fi or who make our double soy lattes do not bring further considerations to bear on whether to give us what we want. They do not consider the appropriateness of our desire for a double soy latte; they do not ask what websites we'll be visiting. We expect them to obey ordinary norms of law and not defraud or deceive, but beyond that we expect them to do as we wish (provided that they can perform the service, and we can pay). There is no distinctive professional ethic for these practices because there is no profession, no deep orientation to a good or set of goods, that gives meaning and purpose to what they do.

Thus, in the provider of services model, the work of physicians becomes demoralized, and its ethic becomes what the philosopher H. Tristram Engelhardt has identified as a "morality of strangers."[4] One does not knowingly do violence to the unconsenting innocent, to be sure. But within the boundaries of law and consent, what is technically possible is ethically permissible. That which is permissible and also desired may even be ethically obligatory. Medical ethics reduces to a set of procedures for negotiating noninterference with patients' wishes to the greatest possible extent. Medicine itself devolves into a powerful set of means to be used to satisfy the preferences and desires of those who are authorized, legally and procedurally, to *choose*.

Among the many consequences of the provider of services model, the following three loom. First, professional authority has steadily eroded. If there is no objective standard or *end* for medicine, physician expertise is merely technical. Thus, instead of exercising the authority of expertise within a sphere constituted by their professional commitments, physicians become increasingly subject to the exercise of power by lobbyists and political advocacy groups. Medical professionals come to work in a highly regulated domain in which the exercise of clinical judgment and prudence is neither possible nor desirable.

It's no surprise, then, that declining professional authority is followed by a second consequence: a crisis of medical morale. Insofar as medicine merely provides desired services, its pretense of moral seriousness is a charade, and its attempts at professionalism are a façade. The practice of medicine is characteristically grueling, with long hours spent under taxing circumstances. Is it surprising that physicians who experience themselves largely as mere functionaries—asked to set aside traditional medical norms, religious convictions, and their best judgment—suffer high rates of burnout?[5]

Finally, when medicine is understood as the provision of healthcare services, the physician's judgment—and particularly the physician's claims of conscience—come to be seen in competition with the fundamental, but minimal, norms of the profession. The exercise of physician conscience is treated as the intrusion of "private" or "personal" concerns into transactions that should be governed by physicians' professional commitment to provide legally permitted services to patients who request those services. Michael and Tracy Balboni note that this artificial separation of the personal and professional leads patients and clinicians to suppress and ignore their moral and spiritual concerns, to the detriments of both.[6] As a result, the medical profession and society at large appear increasingly ready to abandon the idea of the conscientious physician and to use the coercive powers of the profession and the state to compel physicians to participate in practices that violate norms that have guided medical practitioners for millennia.

THE WAY OF MEDICINE

What is our alternative vision for medicine? We call it the *Way of Medicine*. The Way of Medicine offers physicians both a path out of the provider of services model (PSM) and the resources necessary to resist the various political, institutional, and cultural forces that constantly push practitioners and patients to think of their relationship in terms of an economic exchange. We attempt in this book to articulate and defend this Way of Medicine.

Medicine as a Practice

We begin by arguing that medicine is a paradigmatic practice, elevated to a profession because of its social importance, that aims at human health. Health is an objective natural norm for any organism: the well-functioning of that organism as a whole. Human health is also an objective human good: *our* organic well-functioning is an aspect of our human flourishing. Understood in this twofold way, health gives singular purpose to the practice of medicine.

The PSM also concerns itself with health; no one, to our knowledge, denies the importance of health to the practice of medicine. But under the PSM, health is only a subjective and socially constructed concept. Therefore, the norm of "health" is sufficiently malleable to justify pursuing almost any desired bodily condition. In addition, many see health, however defined, as only one among a number of goals toward which medicine might reasonably be aimed. For the PSM, pursuing health is optional.[7]

In contrast, in the Way of Medicine, the good physician orients her practice centrally around the good of health. Physicians need only pursue those aims related to health, and the profession as a whole should, to the extent possible, avoid entanglement with goods other than health—except when necessary to understand and address patients' health-related needs. In detaching from the objective demands of health in favor of a broader and more subjective mandate, the medical profession makes a grave mistake of prudence. Such detachment erodes the grounds for treating medicine as a profession rather than as a technical trade; the professional commitments of medicine are watered down, and physicians find themselves lacking the excellence that is made possible by sustained focus on a single good.

Physicians and other members of the medical profession must also, according to the practice of medicine, resist inducements to act in ways that contradict the good of health. This commitment dates back to Hippocrates and the promise the physician makes in the Hippocratic Oath to "give no deadly potion" nor "cause an abortion" no matter how much the physician is implored to do so.[8] In the Way of Medicine, physicians are always justified in refusing to intentionally damage or destroy the good of health. But this is very different from saying that physicians should avoid any action that even indirectly injures health; the rule of double effect has for centuries helped clinicians practicing the Way of Medicine to discern when they can accept as side effects of health-oriented interventions harms that they should never intend.[9]

The Way of Medicine obviously requires that physicians do more than refuse to damage the good of health. Physicians must devote themselves to that good, not in the abstract but as it bears on their patients' concrete needs. Medical practice is neither a pastime nor merely a career; it is a *profession*, whose members make life-shaping commitments to care for particular vulnerable persons. The patient necessarily occupies a privileged position in the physician's life, as a focal point of his concern and care. At the same time, the physician who practices the Way of Medicine pursues the health of his particular patients while mindful that health is not the only good, nor are his patients the only ones in need.

The Requirements of Practical Reason

The Way of Medicine starts with attention to the kind of practice medicine is and the good toward which medicine aims, but it does not stop there. People who pursue the health of patients must do so in ways that respect the broader demands of ethics. (We use the terms "ethics," "morality," and "practical reason" interchangeably.) Put differently, the practice of medicine has its own integrity, but that integrity depends on and is accountable to the requirements of practical reason.

The requirements of practical reason have been known under a number of names. One is *natural law*. Natural law is not law inscribed in the heavens but rather the practical reason that directs persons to act. C. S. Lewis identified another name, *the Tao*, as a synonym for practical reason and natural law, which he describes as the "source of all value judgments."[10] These various names point to the same reality: practical reason's identification of that which is genuinely good for human beings—that is, conducive to human flourishing—and the corollary implications as to what we should do and how we should live.

What goods contribute to human flourishing? Practical reason identifies several goods as giving human persons fundamental and basic reasons for action: friendship, knowledge, and play are three examples. Human life and health constitute another such good: we are better off, as individuals and in community, if we are alive and healthy. Health is not good only in order to achieve some other purpose; its goodness is what philosophers call *basic*. We can reasonably preserve a life for its own sake; we can reasonably pursue health simply in order to be healthy.

So practical reason gives us the principle that health should be valued and pursued. What are the implications of that principle for the Way of Medicine? Here we find that the internal norms of the practice of medicine are strongly confirmed by what practical reason requires, unlike, say, the internal norms of the practice of torture. Practical reason forbids us to intentionally damage or destroy any basic human goods, including the good of health. Practical reason thus adds to and deepens the norms internal to medical practice, but it does not contradict those norms. In the Way of Medicine, a practitioner focuses on the patient's health but does so while respecting and being guided by the fuller requirements of practical reason.

AN OPEN INVITATION

In this book we invite the reader to join us on a quest to investigate the Way of Medicine. While we write primarily for those who are dissatisfied with the PSM, we welcome any readers with an interest in contemporary healthcare.

We do not intend to divide the medical profession into two starkly distinct camps. We recognize that our description of the PSM may seem like a caricature to some practitioners, who find themselves agreeing fully neither with the PSM nor with our account of the Way of Medicine. These readers may call themselves "providers," but they are devoted to providing quality healthcare and they take seriously the duty to do no harm to their patients' health. Yet they also see much value in respecting patients' choices and providing healthcare services that align with what the patient believes is good for him or her.

In fact, the PSM and the Way of Medicine both operate in the practices of most clinicians—to different extents in different contexts. Few physicians practice consistently within only one or the other, and the two accounts coexist amicably so long as what patients want is for their practitioners to use their best judgment to pursue the patients' health. Most patients do want just that most of the time. But ultimately, as we will show, the two accounts are irreconcilable and the future of medicine will be determined by which one governs the profession.

What might readers who deeply value what the PSM offers gain from learning about the Way of Medicine? At a minimum, they will come to understand what still attracts some of their colleagues to this once regnant, but now contested, vision of medicine as an honorable profession. Even if we fail to win over such readers, we can at least contribute to the promotion of civility and mutual respect among those who disagree.

Still, in this book we speak primarily to those who are disposed to recognize and affirm that human health is a good that medical practitioners can know objectively and pursue conscientiously. The book is primarily for people convinced that some real moral boundaries should never be traversed—for example, physicians should never kill or deliberately harm their patients, even when patients request it. These convictions still run deep in the medical community, but those so convinced inhabit a culture and a profession that have lost the language (and the arguments) to make sense of these eminently reasonable propositions. Without such language, it can be hard for physicians, ethicists, and even patients to find their way. In this state of affairs, for example, we observe physicians who know that they should never kill their patients and are deeply unsettled by medical and societal pressures to the contrary but who have lost the language to talk about how that commitment to life and health is integral to medicine. With respect to such physicians and others, our task is to reintroduce a more fitting vocabulary to make sense of what they already know.

If we succeed, our physician readers will leave this book with tools, concepts, and arguments that help them practice medicine well while enabling them to account for what they are up to *as physicians*. If our argument is sound, such readers' practice of medicine will have a coherence and goodness that others will both admire and want to emulate. Professional bioethicists and healthcare policymakers will also find resources to address some of the most contested ethical issues of our day. Finally, those whom the profession of medicine serves have something to gain, for our book helps identify what *patients* can reasonably expect of medicine.

THE PROVIDER OF SERVICES MODEL IN HISTORICAL CONTEXT

A full history of what we call the provider of services model goes beyond the scope of this book, but Gerald McKenney, in his book *To Relieve the Human Condition*, traces the PSM's roots to the writings of René Descartes and Francis Bacon. Bacon saw in modern science the means to "relieve and benefit the condition of man" by reducing suffering and expanding the realm of human choice, ostensibly noble goals.[11] Unfortunately, as McKenney observes, this imperative to relieve suffering and expand choice finds in contemporary culture no larger framework of meaning in which to discern which suffering should be relieved and which choices should be accommodated. In the resulting moral vacuum, medicine comes to relieve any condition that an individual experiences as a burden; maximizing choice becomes the default.

What McKenney calls "the Baconian project" takes the human body to be without any given purpose or end (telos)—without what Aristotle called a *final cause*. Jeffrey Bishop, in *The Anticipatory*

Corpse, traces out how modern medicine was birthed historically and argues that the loss of a teleological understanding of the body produced a medicine that treats the body as so much matter in motion and death as simply the terminus of that motion.[12] In Bishop's account, contemporary medicine has come to have no purpose except that which is given to it, post hoc, through the choices of those socially empowered to do so—in our era, autonomous individuals. If an individual chooses to use medicine in a certain way—to manipulate their body in some way or even to cause their own death—the choosing itself is taken to make that use of medical technology ethical.

Although McKenney, Bishop, and other critics of contemporary medicine such as H. T. Englehardt and Stanley Hauerwas all have different points of emphasis, each finds this turn toward maximizing choice and minimizing suffering according to the wishes of the patient to impoverish medicine. All urge, in different ways, the restoration of final causality (purpose) to our understanding of life, death, and medical practice. All call for medicine to be situated within an ethical framework in which illness and suffering, and the practices of medicine, are understood against a vision of humans flourishing as the mortal, rational animals that they are. The arguments we make in this book intersect with, diverge from, and are indebted to the work of these and other critics of contemporary medicine. However, our primary task is to articulate and defend our own account, and so we do not trace these intersections, divergences, or debts here at any length.

THE WAY OF MEDICINE AS A TRADITION

We have suggested that what we call the "the Way of Medicine" constitutes the practice of medicine, deepened, corrected, and shaped by the requirements of practical reason. Some readers may be suspicious of this language because they doubt the existence of *the* Way of Medicine. Such skepticism is likely to be heightened insofar as our account invokes the Hippocratic "tradition" of medicine. As Bishop puts the point, "It is indeed odd to think that there has been real continuity between Hippocrates and the medicine of today."[13]

The objection can be extended. Has not medicine always—the skeptic might ask—encompassed arguments, exceptions, contradictions, and confusions? When, if ever, has medicine been characterized by sufficient uniformity—"hegemony," the dubious might say—to justify speaking of *the* Way of Medicine? We take this objection seriously, as uniformity rarely exists with regard to any human activity. Consider a parallel problem with designating something as "traditional." Traditional marriage—for example, a man and woman joined in a permanent and exclusive union—is found at least as often in the breach as in the observance.

Nevertheless, just as the phrase "traditional marriage" identifies a core set of beliefs and practices, adopted by many and constituting a "social imaginary" that could be found deeply embedded within Western culture,[14] so does the "Way of Medicine" designate a core set of beliefs and practices adopted by many and constituting a social imaginary within which doctors and patients have understood much of what has been expected of medicine and its practitioners.

So while the Way of Medicine (like "Hippocratic Medicine") has a somewhat idealized quality to it, it identifies a discernible tradition with characteristic practices along with ideas that make sense of those practices. More important, this tradition gives rise to what thinkers such as Edmund Pellegrino have called the "internal morality of medicine,"[15] whereby the norms that govern physicians *as physicians* emerge from the particular needs to which the practice of medicine responds and the goods toward which the practice aims. The Way of Medicine identifies the "traditional practice" that, as McKenney writes, emphasized health as a "standard of bodily excellence."[16]

Moreover, we do not claim that the internal morality of medicine is self-vindicating. As the example of torture reveals, practices can be unreasonable in themselves—intrinsically contrary to human good and human flourishing. Or, as we observe with respect to medicine, an otherwise reasonable practice can grow corrupt, unreflective, or shallow. So one must engage in critical reflection to discern whether, to what extent, and in what dimensions a practice is in fact reasonable. Such reflection, however, is simply a form of attending to the requirements of practical reason, the natural law, or the Tao.

This task, albeit difficult, is incumbent on us all. We need not, however, attempt the task on our own. Just as the practice of medicine has been deeply shaped by healers such as Hippocrates, Jesus, Maimonides, Avicenna, Hildegard von Bingen, Galen, Thomas Percival, and Dame Cicely Saunders, so have a host of philosophers, theologians, legal scholars, and clinicians given deep consideration to the requirements of practical reason in the medical context. The list would begin with Plato, Aristotle, Augustine, Aquinas, and several of the healers mentioned above, but it would include, and not end with, twentieth-century thinkers such as Edmund Pellegrino, Leon Kass, Alasdair MacIntyre, and John Finnis.[17]

The Way of Medicine does identify a tradition, not understood as an unbroken continuity between the past and the present, but in the sense articulated by MacIntyre, as a "historically extended, socially embodied argument."[18] To our own development of that argument we now turn.

CHAPTER ONE

The Way of Medicine

To help us investigate the Way of Medicine and to clarify how it differs from the provider of services model, we now introduce three patients whose clinical cases we follow throughout the remainder of the book:

Cindy Parker is a twenty-year-old undergraduate student who presents to the student health clinic.

Abe Anderson is a fifty-year-old carpenter who makes an appointment to see a local primary care physician.

Nora Garcia is an eighty-year-old widow with multiple chronic diseases who presents for her quarterly appointment with her geriatrician.

With these patients in mind, we return to our fundamental questions: What is medicine, and what is it for? What can Cindy Parker, Abe Anderson, and Nora Garcia reasonably expect of their physicians? What goods or ends give purpose to the practice of medicine? What does it mean to call medicine a "profession," and how should its nature as a profession structure the life of the one who enters it? Oddly enough, physicians rarely ask themselves these questions, nor do medical educators ask them of their students. But the answers to these questions are central to the Way of Medicine.

By contrast, the provider of services model (PSM) either ignores these questions or denies that they can be answered. The PSM denies that medicine has an end or a purpose that can be known. In the absence of a rational purpose for medicine, the "morality of strangers" stands in: physicians must at least gain consent before intervening upon the body of another. But the morality of strangers declines to take up the question that the Way of Medicine poses as central: what actions are, and what actions are not, essential to, acceptable for, or incompatible with the fundamental purposes of medicine and hence with the profession of the physician?

Principlism, the most prominent ethical framework guiding the PSM, explicitly circumvents the question of what medicine is for. Tom Beauchamp and James Childress chose four principles—beneficence, nonmaleficence, justice, and autonomy—that seemed relevant to the kinds of practices in which medical practitioners typically engage, yet their framework neither specifies nor depends on an account of what those practices are supposed to do. Principlism encourages medical practitioners to apply the principles, and one principle, *beneficence*, tells practitioners to do what benefits their patients. But principlism does not specify what, in fact, benefits patients and so leaves open what benefits medicine should seek.

The PSM seems to lack something that should be at the root of medical practice and ethics. We can hardly ask medical practitioners to make an open-ended commitment to use the powers at their disposal to achieve whatever their patients want, much less whatever the state or another third party demands. In so doing we would ask medical practitioners to divest themselves of their moral agency and responsibility. To practice good medicine, one must first understand what kind of practice medicine is, what it is for, and what difference that makes.

Medicine Is a Practice

Medicine, we propose, is a practice. A *practice*, Alasdair MacIntyre writes, is "any coherent and complex form of socially established cooperative human activity through which goods internal to that form of activity are realized in the course of trying to achieve those standards of excellence which are appropriate to, and partially definitive of, that form of activity, with the result that human powers to achieve excellence, and human conceptions of the ends and goods involved, are systematically extended."[1] A practice is found wherever human persons cooperate in the pursuit of a good, grow in excellence at that pursuit over time, and extend their shared wisdom of the good and excellence in pursuing that good across generations. So described, medicine seems like a paradigmatic practice.

To identify which goods are realized internal to this practice, consider MacIntyre's distinction between internal and external goods. MacIntyre gives the example of a child learning to play chess. He notes that we might encourage a child to play chess by offering the child money, and more money if the child wins. In this way, the child might learn to play chess with some skill. But that would not mean that chess could be described adequately as a skilled activity of a particular sort through which one obtains money. Money is external to chess—it has nothing intrinsically to do with it. Indeed, insofar as the child plays for money (or other goods external to chess), the child, MacIntyre notes, will be motivated to cheat—to contradict "those standards of excellence which are appropriate to, and partially definitive of" chess. In contrast, insofar as the child comes to appreciate and pursue the goods internal to chess, the child will both be motivated to respect those standards and realize the goods found in playing chess to an extent otherwise impossible.

The same is true for many human practices, including farming, music, and medicine. Those who practice medicine can do so with a variety of goods in view, but many of these goods—for example, money and social prestige—have nothing *intrinsically* to do with the practice. One can readily imagine a physician practicing medicine without pay and in a context in which she gains no social prestige. Moreover, insofar as a physician practices medicine for money or prestige, the physician is motivated to ignore medicine's "standards of excellence" if by doing so he gains more of these external benefits. We see this whenever a physician recommends medical interventions because those interventions increase the physician's income. In contrast, insofar as a physician comes to appreciate and pursue the goods internal to medicine, the physician will respect the standards, rules, and norms that make medicine possible, and he will also join other practitioners in developing and extending the practice to realize its internal goods to an ever greater depth. In this way, the practice of medicine has been dramatically developed and extended over time.

The distinction between internal and external goods helps to explain why so many physicians and nurses today are dissatisfied with their work.[2] A physician who practices medicine merely as a job does so for its external, extrinsic benefits. If he can obtain such benefits in a different, less burdensome way, he will. In contrast, the physician who practices medicine as a *calling* works for the benefits or goods that are realized in the work itself—its internal or intrinsic rewards. We suggest that physicians today are burning out and becoming alienated from their work in substantial part because they do not experience their activity as sufficiently aligned with and successful in bringing about the goods internal to medicine.

Several features of medicine follow from the fact that it involves active pursuit of genuine human goods in a cooperative manner through time. For example, medicine requires extensive effort and sustained focus from its practitioners. As a parallel, consider the good realized in professional soccer (football, for our non-American readers). To have any prospect of playing professional soccer, players must train and discipline themselves for many years. Similarly, to have any prospect of becoming an excellent physician, medical trainees must study, train, and discipline themselves for many years. Professional soccer players and physicians both pursue the goods instantiated in their practices with such all-in commitment that they must inevitably forgo other opportunities for human goods. This is not because they believe soccer or medicine is the only activity worth pursuing but because pursuing soccer or medicine is central to their particular vocations.

In soccer and medicine alike, sustained effort and commitment make possible constellations and expressions of the goods that would otherwise remain out of reach—those available to a master but not to a dilettante (and those available to a tradition, but not to a here-today-but-gone-tomorrow pastime). Most of us can enjoy the delights of recreational soccer with a few cooperating friends, a patch of lawn, a ball, and a small window of time. Little commitment is required. But the beautiful game of professional soccer is achieved only because numerous people make extensive commitments in cooperation with one another. Similarly, most of us can bandage a minor wound or nurse a cold, but the commitments of those who cooperate to bring about the practice of medicine make possible entirely different levels of healing. No one who is sick wants a physician who plays at medicine in the way that a physician might play at soccer with his children.

Medicine requires commitments to particular goods, and also to particular persons. Medicine requires, first, commitments to that community of persons whose cooperation makes this social practice possible. The comparison with professional soccer may help again: players, coaches, trainers, owners, managers, referees, and fans all cooperate to bring about professional soccer. They form a community constituted around a shared good and a shared will or commitment toward that good. The members of this community cooperate to mobilize diverse resources and to create structures and institutions that facilitate their further cooperation—FIFA (Fédération Internationale de Football Association), the World Cup, and so on—so that the particular instances of goods brought about by professional soccer might be realized.

Similarly, medicine requires a great deal of cooperation among physicians, nurses, pharmacists, other healthcare practitioners, administrators, educators, and of course, patients. Together they form a community constituted around the goods that medicine seeks and a shared commitment to pursue those goods together. The members of the community of medicine cooperate to mobilize resources and to create structures and institutions that facilitate their further cooperation—through hospitals, clinics, operating rooms, professional schools, and so forth—so that the particular goods brought about by medicine might be realized. Even a minor surgery, to succeed, requires major commitments and cooperation.

Of course, anyone familiar with the institutions of soccer such as FIFA also knows that those institutions can become corrupt, focused on the external rather than the internal goods of the game. When that happens, the institutions become not aids but threats to the practice.

Similarly, the institutions of medicine, from medical schools and hospitals to insurance companies and regulatory bodies, can become obstacles to the practice of medicine and its internal goods. Many of the pressures pushing clinicians to embrace the PSM come from these institutions, which threaten to withhold external goods and even to inflict institutional sanctions against those practitioners who, for example, refuse to cooperate in interventions that they believe contradict the purposes of medicine. We investigate the Way of Medicine not least because doing so is an essential first step toward revitalizing medicine's institutional world.

Within the community of persons whose cooperation makes medicine possible, patients occupy the place of honor, and the most fundamental commitment of practitioners *as practitioners* is to their particular patients. Although the term "profession" is now used widely to refer to any specialized practice requiring study and training, classically the term referred to medicine, the law, and the clergy. Each of these practices responds to a profound human vulnerability, and each entails a singular commitment to and solidarity with those who experience that vulnerability. In the case of the clergy, the vulnerability is that of being estranged or separated from God and the community of the faithful. In the case of the law, the vulnerability is that of being exposed to threats posed by adversaries and the power of the state. And in the case of medicine, the vulnerability is that of being at risk for disease, injury, and death.

In the grip of such vulnerabilities, people need trustworthy advocates to whom they can turn for help. These advocates must be trustworthy, first, because the stakes are high. If a soccer player makes a mistake, his team may lose the game. But if an attorney makes a mistake, his client may spend years behind bars. And if a doctor makes a mistake, her patient may die. Because the stakes are high, those who aspire to the clergy, the law, or medicine typically must undergo long periods of training and apprenticeship before they are authorized as practitioners of their profession.

These advocates must be trustworthy, too, because in order to receive their help, the one in need must entrust himself to the advocate's care, and doing so makes the one in need profoundly vulnerable to the professional herself. The supplicant must entrust herself to the priest by confessing truthfully and submitting to the priest's ministrations. She makes herself vulnerable to the possibility that the priest will divulge what she confesses or use her information for personal gain. The accused must entrust himself to the attorney by permitting her to represent him before the power of the state. He makes himself vulnerable to the possibility that the attorney will collude with the prosecutor to settle the case in a way that minimizes the attorney's work while miscarrying justice. The patient must entrust himself to the physician by submitting to interventions with substantial side effects and risks. He makes himself vulnerable to the possibility that the physician will recommend the intervention that fattens the physician's wallet rather than the one most likely to bring healing to the patient. In all of these cases, the one in need stands in an acute relationship of vulnerability with respect to the professional.

Because of this vulnerability, those who practice one of these three professions must internalize and reliably display the moral commitments that govern that profession. These commitments become, in MacIntyre's terms, rules and standards of excellence without which the practice cannot long continue. The word "profession" initially referred to taking religious vows or otherwise publicly declaring particular beliefs or commitments. At the heart of the professions of the clergy, the law, and medicine is a commitment to the good of the vulnerable. In medicine, this entails a particular kind of solidarity with one's patients—a commitment to them that prescinds from all judgments about a patient's merit and engenders distinctive and substantial obligations toward the patient.

To the question of what kind of activity medicine is, we can now say that it is a paradigmatic *practice*—and to the question of what kind of practice it is, we can say that medicine is a paradigmatic *profession*. Medicine arises not from a need to bring about the greatest good for the greatest number nor in order to satisfy an array of desires, but rather in response to the threats that disease, injury, and death pose to the flourishing of every human being. Medicine's practitioners devote sustained effort and commitment to preserve and restore those goods that are threatened. They do so in cooperation with and commitment to a community of others who also are concerned to preserve and restore these goods and in solidarity with those individuals who need the goods that medicine exists to seek, preserve, and restore.

This gives us a starting place on the Way of Medicine, but we need more. To know what Cindy Parker, Abe Anderson, and Nora Garcia can reasonably expect from their physicians, we still need to know *which* goods medicine is for.

MEDICINE IS FOR HEALTH

Accordingly, we now make a modest proposal: medicine is for *health*. That health is a human good we consider evident; health gives all human beings a reason for action because it offers all human beings something that contributes to their flourishing. So health is *an end* for everyone in their day-to-day life, a point to which we return in chapter 2.

We acknowledge disagreements regarding both what health is and whether health is *the* end of medicine, and we will address these disagreements below. Nevertheless, we take the claim that medicine is for health to be modest because it is so strongly supported by the evidence of authority, is so implicitly affirmed by the practices and commitments of physicians and patients across moral communities, and so aptly addresses the vulnerability that patients experience, thereby undergirding the solidarity and trust that make medicine possible. Let us address each of these points in turn; in so doing, we identify and describe the Way of Medicine.

First, that health is the end of medicine is a proposal supported by the evidence of authority—the considered opinions of wise practitioners of the art for thousands of years. Though not himself a physician, Aristotle thought it axiomatic that medicine is for health. He wrote, "Now, as there are many actions, arts, and sciences, their ends also are many; the end of the medical art is health, that of shipbuilding a vessel, that of strategy victory, that of economics wealth."[3] Aristotle took these claims as starting points for practical reason, as things known immediately by both "the many and the wise." Similarly, the

Hippocratic Oath includes a promise to enter homes only "on behalf of the sick," implying that medicine's fundamental aim is to restore the health that is imperiled in the sick. Countless practitioners of medicine, before and after, have made the patients' health their goal.

Second, the proposal is implicitly affirmed by the practices and commitments of physicians and patients across diverse moral communities, including those who might deny that medicine has any intrinsic purpose. Indeed, implicit agreement that medicine is (at least) for health seems to be a necessary condition for the practice's existence. One could not mobilize the massive social cooperation necessary to sustain a coherent medical profession in the absence of some shared end. Today, medical technologies can be applied toward many different goals—something we consider in more detail throughout the book. For the moment, we note that with respect to many of these goals (e.g., family planning or a timely death), different religious and other moral traditions have long disagreed. If medicine were understood as a practice of pursuing such goals, there would be no shared medical profession any more than there is a shared clergy profession. Different moral communities simply would not cooperate to bring such a profession about.

Virtually everyone agrees, however, that it is good to care for the sick so as to preserve and restore their health. That commitment is central to Judaism, Christianity, Islam, and other world religions, and it is championed equally by those who do not consider themselves religious at all. That commitment resonates with and makes sense of students' longing to be physicians and of physicians' longing to become more fully the physicians they are not yet. Indeed, though physicians, patients, and bioethicists disagree about many things, we have yet to meet colleagues who challenge the notion that one of physicians' central concerns is their patients' health.

Third, the proposal responds aptly to the particular vulnerability that patients face and evokes the specific form of solidarity and commitment that makes medicine the profession it is. Put another way, medicine as oriented toward patients' health addresses a real and significant need of human persons. Edmund Pellegrino and David Thomasma, among others, have argued that the particular form of vulnerability that sickness brings gives us clear direction regarding the *internal morality* of medicine,[4] or what we are calling the Way of Medicine. If we pay attention to the experiences of those who are sick, we find that they need a skilled helper habituated by a resolute commitment to their good insofar as that good involves health. The commitment to seek their patients' health, and to do so in solidarity with the patient as a person, allows those who are sick to entrust themselves to their physicians. Without such trust, physicians cannot do their work. The ethic of medicine—the Way of Medicine—is grounded in these truths.

"WHY ONLY HEALTH?"

Health may be good, and there may be good reasons to make health a primary focus of medicine, but why *only* health? Why not also direct medicine toward any number of other goals, to bring about other states that otherwise reasonable people also desire? It may seem nothing more than incantation to say that medicine by its nature aims at health. Surely medicine, a social construct, has no nature in any deep sense.

We concede a limited point: there is nothing magical about medicine as a social practice that gives it a lock on the good of health and only that good. The particular way in which goods are realized in a practice depends on the structure and history of that practice. Had medicine been organized and pursued in a different fashion, had its history and traditions been different, it might have become a different practice with a different internal good. However, a certain practice did develop whose primary, and even singular, internal good was health. The question now is this: is there a reason to maintain that traditional practice, the practice identified by the Way of Medicine?

We think the answer is Yes but make a further concession: our argument is, in certain respects, a prudential one. We could imagine, in theory, a profession in which physicians aimed at all kinds of goods while also maintaining excellence in preserving and restoring health, and did so while respecting the further requirements of practical reason. We have not, however, seen such a profession realized in fact. Indeed, bringing one about seems prohibitively difficult.

The first problem is one we have already described: without a clear focus on a common recognized good, it is not possible to engender the social commitments and cooperation necessary for an appropriately capacious practice of medicine. Suppose that doctors were thought to be merely powerful wielders of technology, serving the desires of the highest bidder or the demands of the most powerful institution. What reason could we have for trusting such doctors? Indeed, would it not be more reasonable for those who are sick to hold back from entrusting themselves to such "physicians"? Without trust spread broadly across a variety of moral communities, a public profession of medicine will steadily disintegrate into rival camps that use the powers at their disposal to pursue different and ultimately irreconcilable goals.

That is not to say that the Way of Medicine is monolithic; it allows for diverse practices as long as those practices share the pursuit of health. The good of health allows for complexities and ambiguities, and different moral communities will disagree about how and how much to pursue health relative to other goods. They may even disagree on the margins about what health is. A focus on their patients' health, however, allows clinicians and patients even from diverse moral communities to trust one another in pursuing this limited but crucially important shared goal.

Another problem is that of focus and differentiation. Consider again a professional soccer player. If he begins to use his remarkable foot dexterity to kick field goals in US football, and then to dance rumba, and then to compete in mixed martial arts, at some point he becomes not a professional soccer player but a highly skilled user of his feet. As the scope of his footwork expands, the excellence of his soccer playing will likely diminish, and some uses of foot dexterity may come to contradict his commitment to soccer. (For example, kicking another player would conflict with the internal norms of soccer, and kickboxing might result in injuries that cripple his soccer play.) As a result, professional soccer players generally focus on soccer, not on making things happen with their feet. Similarly, insofar as physicians use the technological powers at their disposal to pursue a wide array of outcomes, they necessarily become less expert and skilled at pursuing their patients' health.

Moreover, as we further consider throughout the book, some uses of medical technology not only distract practitioners from their pursuit of their patients' health but come to contradict that pursuit or otherwise violate the requirements of practical reason. Some alleged healthcare services directly destroy health or other basic human goods. Some satisfy wishes for that which is not good. Some undermine the conditions necessary for patients to entrust themselves to clinicians when they are sick. Some services are simply unfair. By detaching from medicine's orientation to health, the PSM sets aside the internal resources practitioners need in order to resist temptations to abuse their medical powers.

History is punctuated with episodes in which medical powers were abused. Tellingly, in each case the commitment to the patient's health was either set aside or directly transgressed. Many readers are familiar with the Tuskegee experiments, in which physicians tracked African American men suffering from syphilis for years without treating them. In that case, doctors set aside concern for the health of their patients in order to use the patients to pursue scientific knowledge. We could similarly consider the medicine of National Socialist Germany, which was in its time the most scientifically accomplished medical system in the world. There, by trading the health of the patient for the "health" of the "Volk" (the nation), German medicine became the instrument of mass torture and murder.[5] Or again, we could look at the eugenics movement in the United States, in which physicians forcibly sterilized thousands of women to realize a dubious vision of "population health."[6] Wherever medicine as a social institution has gone badly wrong, it has ignored or abandoned its commitment to the patient's health in order to harness medicine's powers to achieve other social goals. Keeping the health of the patient as the end of medicine shores up a wall of defense against such abuses.

WHAT IS HEALTH?

Even if you agree that medicine has a purpose and that the purpose is health, it remains necessary to define "health" further, which poses difficulties. Health is a reality of such breadth and depth that it cannot be known with the same precision as mathematical algorithms. Any definition of health will necessarily be incomplete and will allow, at least on the margins, for uncertainty and ambiguity. For some, perhaps particularly for those conditioned to regard scientific knowledge as the highest form of understanding, that health cannot be defined with precision will be deeply unsatisfying. If health cannot be defined with clear margins, of what use is the concept in specifying the purposes of medicine?

We can still know much about health, because it and its absence are intrinsic to human experience, as they are also to the lives of nonhuman animals. Indeed, the fact that diverse and plural cultures all give rise to healing professions testifies to the way health and the absence of health make themselves known as facts of human experience and are accessible to the inquiry of reasonable people. However, in light of the kind of reality health is, we do well to heed Aristotle's admonition that we not demand of a subject matter more certainty than it allows.[7] In that spirit, we start with what seems obvious regarding health, and we draw distinctions where necessary for clarity.

In this task we are deeply indebted to the work of Leon Kass. In the following paragraphs, we articulate and extend certain aspects of Kass's inquiry into the nature of health.[8] Throughout the rest of the book, we consider further what health is by examining health in particular clinical contexts, and we show that the way one defines health dramatically shapes the way one understands physicians' responsibilities.

The Way of Medicine makes two claims about health and *objectivity*. First, health is an objective bodily norm for all living organisms. "Norm" here does not mean a moral norm; rather, living beings have characteristic bodily activities and tendencies, and these activities and tendencies determine what is appropriate—the norm—for them in regard to the well-working of their organic bodies. Hence, there are objective facts about what health is for any organism, and being right or wrong is possible with respect to questions about an organism's health. When organisms display the health-related norm(s) for members of their kind, we can say that they are healthy.

Second, *human* health is an objective *human* good; health is grasped by human agents as worth pursuing. Likewise, such agents grasp that not valuing health would be unreasonable and that states of ill health are to be avoided. Health as a *bodily norm* and health as *good* are related, of course: health could not be objectively good if there were no facts about what health is. But the two forms of objectivity differ: the health of nonhuman organisms is, like human health, an objective bodily norm for those organisms, yet it is not a human good.

The Way of Medicine takes human health to be objective in both senses: knowable in fact and genuinely good. Denial of either claim leads directly to the PSM, for if health either is not real or is not good, patients have no intrinsic reason to choose health rather than other desired states; nor do physicians have any intrinsic reason to make health central to their practice and profession.

Our claim here should not be misunderstood by reference to a particular dispute that characterizes the current philosophy of medicine. Philosophers disagree about whether health is an objective or an evaluative concept; philosophers advocating the former are attracted to naturalistic accounts of health, often based on the notion of statistically normal function.[9] Those who advocate for the latter hold that what we value determines what we consider to be healthy.[10]

Our view differs from both accounts. Against the former, we hold that living beings are genuinely teleologically ordered. As we will discuss below, organisms have characteristic activities that serve their biological life form, and that life form establishes the objective norm for the organisms' healthy functioning, not mere statistical regularities. Against the evaluative view of health, we distinguish between health's being an objective bodily norm and health's being objectively desirable or valuable. Whether an organism is healthy does not depend on whether health is desired or valued. Hence, one can recognize a squirrel's health, as we do below, without incorporating any judgment that the squirrel's health should be pursued or protected.

What, then, does it mean to say that a living being is healthy? What is the health that the medical profession serves? Here we make four points about what health is, then clarify in certain respects what health is not.

First, the domain of health, in its primary meaning, is not that of parts but of *wholes*. When people speak analogically of healthy marriages or healthy communities, they are concerned with those realities as wholes, and the same is true of health in its paradigmatic sense. Health is a matter of what is true of an organism, the living biological whole that in fact precedes, metaphysically and temporally, the healthy differentiation, growth, and development of its parts.

The term "health" can obviously also be applied to parts of the organism, as to a "healthy liver" or a "healthy heart." But such descriptions are still clearly dependent on our understanding of the health of the whole. A liver or heart is recognized as healthy when it is in a state that serves the health of the whole organism. Likewise, the health of the whole organism is more than the sum of the health of its parts. An organism may have all its parts in apparent working order and yet be in ill health. We see this in patients with syndromes of medically unexplained symptoms.[11] Or an organism may have a deficient or absent part and still be in good health, as we see in many patients who have lost a kidney or spleen, even a limb or an eye. Finally, we know from experience that physicians readily sacrifice a part for the health of the whole, as they do when removing a crushed finger or an infected gallbladder. All these truths testify to the primacy of the organism as a whole in thinking about health.

Second, health is associated importantly with *activity*. Kass describes health aptly as the "well-working" of the organism as a whole. This emphasis on activity militates against the forms of reductionism that equate health with static conditions and abstractions, such as lab values in the expected range, clear radiographic studies, and unremarkable physical exams. In being characterized by activity, health resembles courage or strength, which would not exist unless manifest in action — and it is unlike beauty or stature. Activity does not imply constant movement, of course; thinking, resting, and sleeping are all activities that require and display health. For humans, each is an essential aspect of the well-working of the whole.

Third, the health of an organism and its health activity must be judged, to a certain extent, with sensitivity to the organism's context and state of development. The health of a thirty-year-old woman differs from the health of a thirty-year-old man, and the health of both differs from the health of a ten-year-old of either sex. A healthy ninety-year-old experiences extensive diminishments of health relative to a typical twenty-year-old, yet we can still distinguish between a healthy and an unhealthy ninety-year-old. Similarly, what it means for a person who has a conspicuous disability to be healthy differs from the perception of health of a person who does not.[12]

These differences, present within the population of a species, are more pronounced between species. Hence, our fourth point is that health is species-specific. The health of a dolphin differs markedly from that of a squirrel. The health of both is manifest in the activities they perform *as the sorts of organisms they are.* Being different kinds of organisms, with different natures, their health is different, but in each case we can still speak of the well-working of the organism as a whole. Thus, no one would suspect a squirrel to be in ill health simply because it cannot swim at high speeds under water. And no one would suspect that a dolphin is ill because it cannot climb trees. The signs, expressions, and realizations of health vary from species to species. Human health is more complex because the characteristic activities of healthy human beings are more varied and diverse than those of other organisms. This complexity makes it difficult in some cases to make judgments about health and how to pursue it, as subsequent chapters show.

Do all of these complexities indicate that health is merely a subjective notion, merely a socially constructed concept? They do not. Something can be relative in certain respects while still being objective. Health is objective if there are matters of fact concerning whether some individual organism is healthy, but to discern such matters of fact, one must recognize truths that are relative to that organism's species, stage of life, and particular circumstances. Indeed, health can be subjective in certain respects while still being objective: a clinician may be unable to find anything objectively wrong, but we believe (with Kass) that if the individual sincerely believes she is unhealthy, then to that extent she is. More investigation may be called for in order to determine, if possible, what has gone wrong, but individuals do have a certain epistemic authority in determining whether they are unhealthy.

Health can easily be confused with proximate or related concepts. Health is not the same, for example, as having the least possible risk of future injury, illness, or death. Playing soccer professionally requires a high degree of health but also risks injuries that could be avoided by refusing to play soccer. It does not follow that standing on the sidelines displays greater health than does playing in the game. Similarly, health makes pregnancy possible, while pregnancy also poses risks to health. One who is sterile does not display greater health, however, than one who is capable of pregnancy.

Nor is health the absence of suffering. It is true that physicians have always prioritized relief of suffering. "To cure sometimes, to relieve often, to comfort always," the maxim goes. Poor health is, of course, suffered, and many conditions that diminish health also induce pain and other symptoms that elicit suffering. Yet we also could draw up a long list of conditions people suffer that may affect their health but are not themselves signs of the absence of health. Those who are poor suffer want of finances, and those who lose loved ones suffer heartbreak, to give just two examples. Distinguishing suffering from health has decisive implications for medical ethics, as we note throughout the book. To foreshadow a bit, we observe that some people today, insofar as their experience goes, *suffer* the conditions of having male genitals, small breasts, or short height, or even being alive. If physicians equate health with the absence of suffering, they will try to relieve these and other conditions. This hubristic aspiration leads physicians, in the words of McKenny, "to relieve the human condition."[13]

The distinction between suffering and ill health raises an important question: what about mental health?[14] The challenge is to define "mental health" so that it includes the well-working of an organism's mental and psychological capacities, but it does not expand to require the absence of suffering we just described, nor happiness, nor the satisfaction of every desire. On one end of a spectrum are conditions that seem clearly to represent deficits in mental health: schizophrenia or catatonic depression, to give two examples. On the other end of this spectrum we find sadness, anxiety, grief, or rambunctiousness that are often described as mental and behavioral illnesses but do not clearly display a deficiency of one's health. Often it is not possible to draw a bright line between conditions that display ill health and those that do not. Making these distinctions requires both good clinical judgment and the humility to recognize the limits of such judgment. What medicine should pursue is the mental capacity that makes it possible to experience happiness, sadness, and other emotions in the way that humans experience them when they are well-working, and to make choices and behave in ways that humans are capable of when they are well-working. Medicine oriented to health will not seek to bring about a particular emotional state or a particular set of choices and behaviors as such. By analogy, medicine would seek to preserve or restore the capacity that makes it possible to play a musical instrument, not to determine which notes are played or to ensure that the music remains in a major key.

Finally, although we have noted that the state of health is also objectively desirable, and hence an aspect of human flourishing, the state of being healthy does not encompass all that goes into human flourishing. The World Health Organization errs when it defines health as "a state of complete physical, mental, and social well-being."[15] A related error is made by the agrarian poet and social critic Wendell Berry, whose work emphasizes that human beings flourish only in community. Berry defines health as *membership* and argues that the smallest unit of health should be the community; thus, "to speak of the health of an isolated individual is a contradiction in terms."[16] Such accounts, though admirable as critiques of reductionism and individualism, problematically raise health above other human goods, making health not merely one human good but the state of human flourishing that encapsulates all human goods. If the end of medicine is health so understood—if medicine's purpose is to bring about the fullness of life, the Hebrew concept of "shalom,"[17] the World Health Organization's vision of complete well-being, or even Berry's vision of membership—it seems that physicians have a wide-open mandate. All is their responsibility, all their domain.

Health so understood is not useful for guiding medical practice. Imagine a man who says that he is going to see his physician because he recognizes that he has an unhealthy relationship with his neighbor or he wants to work on getting his finances into better shape. When terms for health are expanded to encompass all aspects of human well-being, the term may inspire but it no longer proves useful, especially not for naming the thing that medicine is for.

According to the Way of Medicine, health is the end or purpose of medicine, the principal goal that medicine seeks, the principal good that is realized internal to medicine's practice. But "health" here is meant in a limited, circumscribed, and embodied sense: what Kass describes as "the well-working of the organism as a whole," realized and manifested in the characteristic activities of the living body in accordance with its species-specific life-form.[18] We believe this account captures the primary meaning of health. Health so understood is also a good that can be pursued for its own sake as one—but only one—constitutive aspect of human flourishing. It is additionally, of course, a condition for the possibility of pursuing other human goods. According to the Way of Medicine, human health understood in these two dimensions—as an objective bodily norm and as an objective human good—grounds medical practice and the medical profession: it is *the* end that takes precedence over others in the practice of medicine, one that is not to be abandoned or violated by those who profess a vocational commitment to it.

Their health, therefore, is what Cindy, Abe, and Nora can reasonably expect will form the center of their relationships with all health-care professionals through all stages of their lives.

CHAPTER TWO

The Requirements
of Practical Reason

Having argued that medicine is for a patient's health, we now consider how medicine's pursuit of the patient's health depends on and is accountable to ethics: the broader requirements of practical reason. The questions that concern us throughout this book are *practical*. They concern action—not action considered impersonally from a spectator's point of view but action considered personally from the standpoint of one who must decide what to do. Practical reason considers questions about particular actions as well as lives as a whole. Humans rightly ask not only "What should I do?" but also "How should I live?" And "What *kind of person* should I be?"

Members of the medical profession clearly need to ask both kinds of practical questions. With respect to particular *actions*, the questions include the following:

- Should I inform this patient of the terminal condition she has, even though it might seem to do no good and might even distress her and cause her suffering?
- Is it permissible to counsel or provide contraceptives or abortion to those who seek to avoid or end unwanted pregnancies?
- Must I respect this patient's wishes that I not provide further nutrition or hydration, that I provide sedation to the point of unconsciousness to alleviate her anxiety, or . . . ?

The medical professional's life is filled with such questions, and the medical practitioner needs an adequate framework for thinking about how best to answer them.

With respect to questions about lives as a whole, the questions include these:

- What sort of doctor [or nurse or therapist] should I be?
- What are the fundamental commitments of my profession around which I must orient my life?
- What sorts of virtues must I have, and how must I discipline my mind, will, and emotions in order to become and remain a good practitioner of medicine?
- How does being a health-care practitioner fit into my other life-shaping commitments, including my commitments to family, to neighbor, and to God? Are these parts of my life walled off from one another? If not, which should take priority, and how should conflicts be negotiated when they arise?

These questions involve how a person should live, and they cannot be answered solely by thinking about the practice of medicine and its internal good, for they concern the relationship of that practice and its good to the other practices, goods, and values in a person's life.

The practice of thinking critically about all of these questions and subjecting the possible answers to reflection and scrutiny is that part of philosophy that can be called ethics, or *practical ethics*. Aristotle kept the practical nature of ethics squarely in focus when he composed his *Nicomachean Ethics*.[1] Engaging in ethics, he wrote, is for the sake of taking action. Some philosophers focus primarily on theoretical questions regarding ethics—for example, questions about the meaning of moral language—but in this book we approach ethics practically, as Aristotle did.

Our understanding of practical ethics is deeply shaped by the tradition of natural law ethics. There are many distortions and abuses of natural law reasoning, particularly those that have defended an unjust arrangement of institutional and social power as "natural" or as expressing the "law of nature." These are not what we mean by a natural law ethics. Rather, a natural law ethics is an attempt to discover the deepest practical principles of human flourishing and to work out the implications of those principles in norms for concrete action. These principles and norms are what we identify as the requirements of practical reason—that which practical reason prescribes when functioning properly. We will argue that this natural law approach to ethics is superior to consequentialist, deontological, and principlist approaches with respect to both moral decision-making in general and medical decision-making in particular.

HUMAN ACTION AND HUMAN GOODS

Let us start with questions about action: Why do we ever act at all? Why not simply *be*, resting in our own personal existence without strain or effort? Surely part of the answer is that human beings in many important respects exist as beings who are "not yet fully formed," who can and must shape themselves by choice and action in order to become more fully what they are capable of being.

No one comes into existence already married, for example, and no one comes into existence already a doctor. Even upon reaching these states, no one is "all done" being either married or a doctor. Rather, being married or being a doctor requires choices and actions that build up our existence as married persons or doctors, fulfilling potentials that we had. But potentials for what? To what does reason direct us? Practical reason's most fundamental principles direct us toward *human flourishing*.

What does "flourishing" mean? Sometimes people talk about "happiness" or "joy" as synonyms for flourishing, but these words can mislead: happiness can be taken as a state of simply feeling good, and joy can be thought of as experienced only momentarily (even if frequently). In contrast, by *"flourishing"* we mean a state of being truly well off as human beings, and sometimes what feels good does *not* makes us truly well off. Moreover, being well off as a human being is something that characterizes a life over time, not just isolated moments. So neither "happiness" nor "joy" captures fully the notion of flourishing, though happiness and joy accompany flourishing in some measure.

Nor is flourishing a self-centered notion, as happiness sometimes is. Human beings are well off and flourish only in community, in relationships with one another, as Wendell Berry reminds us. This point is central in considering the doctor-patient relationship and the importance of patients' relationships to their families. In this way and others, the conception of flourishing we advance differs significantly from what some thinkers have called the self-expressive individualist model of happiness. At its worst, the latter model urges, "If it feels good, do it," reducing human action to expressions of undisciplined self-interest.

In contrast, practical reason begins with human goods. Human action is always oriented toward something perceived as beneficial or good, even when that perception is mistaken. We act for the sake of bringing about something that promises us or others like us some benefit, and this is where we find the foundations of all practical thought: in basic goods that are intrinsic aspects of human well-being or flourishing.

By using "basic" and "intrinsic," we are distinguishing the goods at the foundations of ethics from others that are only instrumental and derivative. Consider the goods of money and medicine. These goods are good only insofar as they promise to bring about something else that is desired. But practical reason starts with those goods that are desirable in themselves for their own sake, because they themselves make all human beings better off and contribute to their flourishing. Basic goods include life and health,[2] knowledge, aesthetic experience, friendship, integrity, religion, and marriage.[3] Each of these particular goods benefits people in unique and irreducible ways. The way we flourish as human beings in attaining knowledge differs from the way we flourish in attaining health. Human flourishing is not reducible to one of these goods, and so, as we will see, a life characterized by flourishing requires some ordering principle within it.

Even bad decisions and lives guided by evil are typically directed at real and basic human goods. Consider again the Tuskegee scandal. This decades-long experiment was a terrible failure of medical morality, yet it was driven by interest in two goods we consider basic: knowledge and health. This presents an essential concern of ethics: how do we get from awareness of the basic goods of human action to making moral decisions in pursuing those goods?

CONSEQUENTIALISM

One answer that many philosophers have defended is that we should maximize goods when making moral decisions.[4] In maximizing, one accounts for all the beings who will be affected by an action, and, as Jeremy Bentham asserted, one promotes the greatest good for the greatest number. Bentham was the founder of the view called *utilitarianism*; utilitarians thought that the good to be maximized was pleasure. Other utilitarian thinkers take different views of what is to be maximized, but we refer to all views of this sort as *consequentialist*, for they all take the goodness or badness of consequences as the primary consideration in making moral judgments.

We have argued elsewhere, at greater length, against consequentialism, and so a few remarks will suffice here.[5] First, consequentialism has at least surface problems with the concepts of justice and rights. Justice and rights seem to be "trumps" against attempts to maximize goodness when that maximization would be unfair to some or would violate basic human rights—for example, threatening persons with enslavement or torture. Second, consequentialism presents significant problems in its demand that we consider all of the consequences that follow from our actions. Our knowledge of such consequences is limited, and that which would fail to maximize consequences in the short term might bear unforeseen but beneficial fruits over time.

The third and most important point to make about consequentialism, and specifically about maximization, is that it cannot work even if consequences could be foreseen reliably, because instances of the goods that are fundamental aspects of human well-being and flourishing cannot themselves be weighed against one another rationally. For example, what do person A's long-term health and person B's long-term knowledge have in common that would provide a metric by which we could say that there is *greater goodness* in A's health or B's knowledge? Health and knowledge are different goods, and these persons are different persons. The options at stake in a decision to, for example, pursue an experiment at the cost of A's health or desist at the cost of B's knowledge seem *incommensurable*—they do not have a common measure of goodness between them that would make maximization possible. Nor are the values of persons' lives commensurable: each person's life is uniquely and immeasurably valuable. We cannot say without qualification, therefore, that this one person should be sacrificed in order to save those two, three, or twelve.

Indeed, even options that a single good generates do not seem genuinely commensurable. Medical professionals and patients regularly face options in which different health benefits are offered, usually accompanied by differing health burdens. A proposed course of surgery plus radiation treatment might offer a patient hope of a longer life, albeit with considerable side effects such as nausea, pain, and reduced energy. A proposed watchful waiting approach might offer hope of preserved energy, appetite, and freedom from disabling pain, albeit with considerable risk of dying sooner. Does one of these options offer all the good of the other plus more? If it did, there would be no need for choice; we would be irrational not to take the greater good. But choice is required. The benefits and burdens of each option differ, and they allow for no common scale of goodness or value through which to resolve one's deliberation.

THE FIRST MORAL PRINCIPLE

What, then, should characterize our relationship to those goods that are basic aspects of all human beings' flourishing? How can we make upright choices when faced with options that involve incommensurable goods and persons? The basic norm would seem to be as follows: *in acting and willing, always be fully open to the goodness of the goods and to the persons for whom those goods are good.* This seems to be a demand of reason, and hence a requirement of practical reason. Practical reason orients us to the goods as we consider what to do, and reason recognizes those goods as giving a point to what we do. Reason, then, requires that we not close ourselves off to goods and persons.

First, let's consider how emotion or prejudice might lead us to be less than fully open to human goods or persons. Consider a situation in which we very much want to experience the benefits of a particular good. This good especially appeals to us or plays an important role in our own or our loved ones' lives. All humans respond more immediately, on some occasions, to some goods rather than others. For example, a particular opportunity to obtain knowledge (say, by reading a book) may seem tedious by comparison with a desirable opportunity for play. On some occasions, options are not merely tedious but painful—going through surgery, working through a difficult rehabilitation, or telling a patient an unpleasant truth. On still other occasions, the good at stake seems of overwhelming importance because it is under threat: our life, for instance—or our career, our family, our religion, and so on.

These responses are understandable, but under the influence of emotion, we sometimes make choices that are not fully open to all goods but instead privilege one or another in an unreasonable way. We might simply choose directly against one good for the sake of another: we deliberately inflict harm on one person for the sake of benefiting someone else, or we deliberately damage one instance of a basic good for the sake of another. Such actions make sense only if goods and good options are weighable. Harming or destroying a good for the sake of some other good makes sense only if that other good is a greater good. Yet the notion of "greater good" is out of place in speaking of basic goods.

Thus, a norm emerges from consideration of the rational requirement of openness to all goods: one should never directly damage or destroy one instance of a basic good for the sake of some other or "greater" good. Of course, one should not damage or destroy an instance of a basic good out of hostility, either, whether hostility toward that good or toward the person experiencing the good. So this norm can be broadened: *one should never, for any reason, directly damage or destroy an instance of a basic human good.* This norm is echoed in the Way of Medicine's millennia-old commitment to do no (intentional) harm. We might say that practitioners of the Way have seen in the domain of medicine and the basic good of human health a genuine requirement of practical reason, and they have sought to respect that requirement in the norms of their practice.

Another requirement of reason has a justification similar to the previous one. Suppose we are attached not just to some good but to some person. Such attachment is often quite reasonable: we have attachments to our children, spouse, and parents, as well as to our neighborhood, workplace, and church. These attachments play a legitimate role in our moral deliberations. Sometimes, however, our emotions lead us to privilege some persons over others in ways that are unreasonable. For example, we allow our daughter to take a greater share of something than the other children, because she is ours; maybe we cheat in our effort to get into medical school, thus privileging ourselves over others who are more qualified. How can we test for this kind of arbitrary privileging in our personal attachments?

One traditional test is the Golden Rule: do unto others as you would have them do unto you. When our privileging diminishes others in such a way that we would resent such privileging were we on the receiving end, we have reason to think that we are acting unreasonably, arbitrarily, and unfairly. Similarly, when we treat others less well than we would expect our loved ones to be treated, we are again acting unfairly. A norm of fairness, clearly violated in the Tuskegee experiments, emerges from the requirement to be open to the goods in all persons.

Of course, sometimes our commitments require that we give some people special treatment: physicians' commitments to their patients, for example, create a special space in their lives for those patients and their needs. But this seems clearly fair: everyone has reason to accept the possibility of such special commitments, for without them, there could be no medical profession, no doctor-patient relationships, none of the benefits that come from a doctor's special knowledge and even her friendship with her patients.

At the same time, the Golden Rule—the norm of fairness—does chasten even such commitments to patients. Physicians will find some patients more pleasant or attractive than others, as does any teacher with respect to her students. When those feelings are allowed to unduly shape medical practice or teaching, a key requirement of practical reason has been violated. To choose one visible example, consider the case of Jahi McMath, an African American teenager in Oakland who was diagnosed as brain dead following a terrible complication of a minor surgery. As described in the *New Yorker*, biases of race and class appear to have affected how medical professionals and professional ethicists treated Jahi and her family.[6] Insofar as that is true, such treatment was unfair and did not adequately meet the requirements of practical reason.

PRINCIPLISM AND KANTIAN ETHICS

Medical ethics as a field emerged in the twentieth century partially in response to abuses and scandals in the medical profession and partially because the profession seemed insufficiently self-critical with respect to its ethical commitments. The emergence of new medical technologies added fuel to the fire by generating dilemmas that seemed to call for new forms of deliberation. "The Belmont Report," issued by the National Commission for the Protection of Human Subjects of Biomedical and Behavioral Research, identified three principles to govern moral action in biomedical research: respect for persons, beneficence, and justice.[7] Within a few years, Thomas Beauchamp, a philosopher and original member of the commission, and James Childress, a theologian, had revised and expanded these to four principles to govern the practice of medicine: autonomy, beneficence, nonmaleficence, and justice.[8]

Beauchamp argued that what has come to be called *principlism* marked an important advance in bioethics. Doctors, he explained, had been attending only to beneficence and nonmaleficence—to doing good and avoiding evil—and so had come to overlook abuses of patient autonomy, as when patients were treated without their consent, and abuses of justice, as when vulnerable populations such as disabled children or poor black sharecroppers were exploited as research subjects. Principlism not only responded to insufficient self-reflection, expanding medical technologies, and abuses of medical ethics; it also seemed to overcome an intractable dispute between two competing schools of ethical thought: consequentialism (discussed above) and Kantian deontology (discussed below). Consequentialists and Kantians espouse different and irreconcilable first principles, but Beauchamp and Childress discovered that even persons with radically different moral foundations could agree on so-called mid-level principles. Principlism appeared to advance bioethics by providing a common approach, even if it eschewed moral foundations.

Interestingly, a number of competing approaches arising in response to principlism also avoided first principles. Bernard Gert and K. Danner Clouser put forward a rule-based approach similar in many respects to principlism, and Albert Jonsen and Stephen Toulmin advocated an approach based on casuistry that looked at paradigm cases and worked by analogy from there to uncertain cases. Theorists including Edmund Pellegrino and David Thomasma defended approaches centered on the virtues that medical professionals should have.[9]

These approaches have varying strengths and weaknesses, but all (with the possible exception of Pellegrino and Thomasma's) share an opposition to foundationalism, to beginning from first principles from which norms (or rules, principles, or even virtues) are derived. Instead, these approaches typically work with the concept of *reflective equilibrium*, which involves moving back and forth between general and abstract norms and concepts, on the one hand, and the features of particular cases, on the other. Many people, especially those engaging in actual clinical practice and not operating "by theory," have found these reflective equilibrium-based approaches refreshingly practical. Notwithstanding their flexibility and practicality, in our view these approaches fail insofar as they lack moral absolutes.

Note that we are not claiming that one right answer always exists for everyone and everybody. In very many circumstances, various options are *all* morally permissible. In many other circumstances, one cannot determine what should be done without taking into account the personal character, choices, commitments, and features of the agents in the situation. No impersonal algorithm can churn out the right answer for everyone in a similar situation. Accordingly, one needs the virtue of prudence, along with a willingness and ability to reflect on one's particular situation, in order to arrive at reasonable decisions.

So in speaking of moral absolutes, we do not claim that some one-size-fits-all model should settle all moral questions, but we do claim that some actions *never* should be performed, regardless of the circumstances. Historically, the medical profession has acknowledged such moral absolutes. The Hippocratic tradition, for example, held that physicians should never kill, and this norm that arose in a pagan society has been affirmed in Jewish, Christian, and Muslim cultures. It is hard to see how ethical approaches that have no foundations can support this or other absolute norms. Rather, nonfoundationalist approaches, particularly principlism, commit to balancing or weighing competing principles in different circumstances based on the features of each individual case. But if all principles (or rules, cases, or virtues) may be weighed against one another, and if all are subject to possible revision in light of a particular circumstance, none are absolute. Nothing, that is, can be ruled out altogether before considering the circumstances.[10] Thus the seemingly absolute demands of human rights—against acts such as rape, torture, and killing the innocent—cannot be absolute after all within a framework like principlism. In contrast, our approach leaves room for these and other moral absolutes.

A related difficulty with principlism and many of its descendants is that they give no account of what is *good*.[11] Consider autonomy, the first of the four principles. Respect for autonomy is essential in medicine, but why? What good or goods does respect for autonomy serve? Similar questions arise with respect to beneficence and nonmaleficence. If we are to do good and avoid doing evil, we must know what is good. Even justice requires an account of what is good, insofar as justice often involves rightly distributing goods and is premised on concern for the good of others.

In this light, we need to unearth the foundations of ethics and seek an account of what is truly good. In our proposal regarding the basic goods, we attempt to provide the deeper content necessary to make sense of Beauchamp's and Childress's midlevel principles, the casuistry of Jonsen and Toulmin, and so on. Moreover, these basic goods allow us to identify moral absolutes, actions that should never be taken precisely because they involve acting contrary to a basic good. Such actions violate the principles of beneficence and nonmaleficence by contradicting genuine goods and thereby human flourishing. They violate justice because they disregard the good of another.

Similar points can be made about Kantian ethics. In his attempt to drill down to the foundations of morality, Immanuel Kant held that a "categorical imperative" was an absolute prescription of reason and that *the* categorical imperative could be formulated as follows: "Act in such a way that you treat humanity, whether in your own person or in the person of another, always at the same time as an end and never simply as a means."[12] Put another way, Kant saw the foundation of ethics as resting on a principle of respect for persons. Human beings are never to be treated as mere things—disposable or usable for others' purposes—but rather must be treated as beings of noncontingent, immeasurable worth. Kant's approach has obvious merits when we consider experiments performed on the unconsenting and unsuspecting not for their own benefit but to serve others' interests. But Kant also left out of consideration, quite deliberately, concern for human good. In Kant we find a prototype of what later came to be described as prioritizing the right over the good, a feature of Kantianism that prevents one from determining the content of what respect for persons requires.

This content-thin feature of Kantianism is especially conspicuous in the work of thinkers who reduce respect for persons to respect for persons' autonomy. What does respect for another as a person mean? It means, on one account, respecting another's capacity to respond to human reasons. In that construal, we violate the categorical imperative when we act toward another without giving reasons and obtaining acquiescence in those reasons—in other words, when we act without the other's informed consent.

But this account of respect also seems thin, reduced to respecting what the other happens to want. Without an account of what is genuinely good for human beings, we have no objective standard against which to judge whether a reason is good—whether, for example, what a patient wants aligns with or contradicts her genuine welfare or flourishing. We are not here advocating overriding a patient's refusal; there are good reasons to respect and insist on patient consent. Nevertheless, if the doctor is to give good reasons, and if the patient is to consider and make an autonomous decision on the basis of those reasons, both parties must have access to some standard for good reason. That standard, we argue, is found in the basic goods and in openness to all such goods in all persons.

The inheritors of the right-is-prior-to-the-good maxim have played another important role in the emergence of the provider of services model (PSM), specifically in its development as a matter of politics. Followers of the political philosopher John Rawls have used that maxim, as well as Kantian thought about reasons and respect for persons more broadly, to argue that only "public" reasons are legitimate for public deliberations and debate.[13] That view has radical consequences for the role of religion in bioethics, especially in bioethics as it plays itself out in political debate, deliberation, legislation, and adjudication. The Rawlsian emphasis on public reason threatens to push religious considerations out of the public sphere—with respect not only to politics but also to the public practice of medicine. Medical professionals, in a Rawlsian model, must resist the influence of religious reasons on their professional deliberations and clinical practices. We assess and criticize this claim in our final chapter, when we take up conscience and medical ethics. But in this chapter the topic of religion raises a somewhat different though ultimately related issue. Religion clearly plays an ordering role in some agents' lives, a role that could be described as vocational; medicine also seems to play such a role.

VOCATION

At the foundation of ethics we find basic human goods that are never to be violated. But any ethic concerned with human flourishing needs more than prohibitions; it also needs an ethic of *pursuing* human goods.

According to practical reason, how should this pursuit of human goods be organized? Why organize at all? Why not simply pursue human goods serially, acting for the sake of this good now, of that good then, in accordance with whatever seems appropriate and desirable in each situation? This question almost answers itself. A life characterized by pursuing goods in such a serial manner, without organization or structure, will inevitably be shallow and chaotic in ways detrimental to human flourishing.

Consider, for example, the following sorts of difficulties. First, such a life could not achieve excellence at anything. Many instances of basic goods can be realized only through sustained effort and commitment. Although one can learn new things from social media and play at the guitar in one's spare time, one cannot realize the good of knowledge available to a first-rate scholar without years of study or the goods of play and aesthetic experience available to a professional guitarist without years of practice. Similarly, a physician cannot bring about her patients' health without first committing to decades of study, practice, and work. Sustained commitments are necessary to realize basic goods in any depth.

Second, achieving basic goods often requires making commitments to other persons. In many cases, pursuit of a good is best organized socially. One cannot become a doctor or a philosopher, for example, without cooperating with other persons. Moreover, some goods are social by nature: no one flourishes, for example, without the good of friendship, yet friendship involves committed relationships with other persons. Achieving basic goods requires a settled will to work with and for others.

Third, once one starts to make commitments—to a profession, a spouse, a church, and so on—one quickly encounters apparent conflicts between these commitments. Therefore, one must put one's commitments in order to be genuinely oriented to human flourishing. We need something like a rational life plan for our actions and lives.

Even so, the idea of a rational life plan fails to capture adequately what we are addressing. First, the language "rational life plan" seems to suggest that we have the power, through a firm will and expert planning, to author our lives as we see fit, but this surely is an error. In some sense, humans are the authors of their own lives through their choices, commitments, and actions. Yet people face in life much more than what we choose or will. Things happen to us, and a good life depends on responding well to such happenings and integrating what has happened *into* the order of our lives. Rarely can we do so without revising our assumptions about that order.

The notion of a rational life plan is less than satisfying for a second reason: it fails to capture the way in which many people believe themselves to have been called to the particular shape of their lives in a manner beyond their control. The concept of calling—a synonym of "vocation"—has roots in traditional Christianity, in which God calls human persons to various and distinct lives of good works, marking out their good deeds in advance for them. In this understanding, one may be called to be a doctor, rather than simply deciding to be one, and in accepting the call, one is constituting oneself in the deepest way not simply as a doctor but also as a person responsive to and responsible before God.

Interestingly, although the concept of calling has roots in Christianity, today most US physicians, regardless of their religious affiliations, use the term to describe their practice of medicine. Indeed, even among physicians who say they have no religion, and among those who say they never attend religious services, more than half agree with the statement "For me, the practice of medicine is a calling."[14]

This result should not surprise us in light of the kind of good that health is. Like knowledge or friendship, health transcends any one person's desires or capacities. Health is good for all human beings, regardless of whether they want it. Moreover, health is a good of such breadth and depth that one can pursue it in countless different ways and explore its meaning and potential for all time. What's more, while it is incommensurable with all other goods, health nevertheless serves as a necessary condition for the pursuit of all other goods. And so, faced with such a good, even nonreligious persons may find that this good calls out to them, inviting them to a lifetime of service. In this sense, physicians might rightly describe their practice of medicine as part of their calling or vocation.

Vocations shape the lives of individuals in at least two important ways. First, vocational commitments generate new obligations. When spouses marry, they commit to one another and to a form of life that generates new obligations for each of them: toward one another as well as toward any children who might result from their marriage. When a student freely makes a vocational commitment to practice medicine rather than teaching philosophy, that commitment requires an array of further commitments and obligations (e.g., to complete premedical courses, take the MCAT, and apply to medical school). A vocational commitment serves in some ways as a promissory obligation, binding an agent voluntarily in a way that she would not otherwise have been bound.

But vocational commitments also free agents from other obligations. A person's vocational commitments to his own children create obligations to care for them that result in having lesser obligations to care for other people's children. A physician's obligations to her profession and to the persons to whom she has obligations within that profession (especially her patients) similarly require her to dedicate her time and effort to meet the needs of those persons, not just any person or every person. Here again, vocational commitments are like promises that, by creating specific obligations, free persons up from more general and unspecified demands that might have been placed on them.

How does one discern one's vocation? Obviously, many people are drawn to the prospect of being a doctor. Equally obvious, however, is that among these many are not "called" per se. How should a person think about whether she is called to this profession or not?

In one way, the answer to this question depends on everything we say through the rest of this book. If we correctly assess what being a doctor means, what the practice of medicine is for, and what moral norms healthcare professionals should abide by, a person should not commit to the medical profession unless she can willingly and enthusiastically embrace and internalize the Way of Medicine. More specifically, she shouldn't become a doctor unless she is willing to embrace the norm of never intending to damage the health of any person. In our approach, one who thinks of her mission as primarily to minimize suffering, even by killing if necessary, does not understand the vocation of medicine and so cannot be called to it in this case.

More generally, though, one can say that vocational commitments should be guided by ability, interest, opportunity, and need. Ability is obvious. No one can become a good surgeon without developing some requisite skills, and some lack the capacity, realistically, to develop those skills. Moreover, "skills" are not enough; they must be joined to dispositions that some people will struggle to develop. A physician in training who dislikes people is in the wrong line of work. The same is true of a pediatrician who finds children tedious, an aspiring surgeon who recoils at the sight of blood, or any medical student or physician motivated primarily by money. The medical profession rightly plays gatekeeper with regard to these skills and dispositions, rejecting many applications to medical school or residency training. But the profession's gatekeeping role cannot substitute entirely for the scrutiny that an individual should give to her own deliberations about whether she has the ability to fulfill the requirements of particular line of work. If she does not, she has reason to believe that she is not called to that line of work.

What about interest? Is it possible to devote one's life to a practice or profession in which one has little interest? Yes, clearly. Some have no option but to do work in which they have little interest. But other things being equal, one's interests and passions serve as helpful guides as to what one is called to do. Suppose an individual has gifts that make him capable of becoming either a fine surgeon or a fine musician, and he is passionate about music but indifferent to medicine. Then, it seems to us, despite some obvious economic trade-offs, that a life in music might be more appropriate for that individual. Passion, however, is not enough. In our culture we frequently hear outrageously talented athletes or other performers say, "You can do anything you put your mind to." No, you cannot. That caveat notwithstanding, human beings are not simply rational; we are also emotional, and the basic good of integrity is enriched in our lives when reason, choice, action, and emotion all harmonize with one another. So attending to one's emotions, passions, likes, and dislikes is an important part of discerning one's vocation.

Third comes opportunity. Recall that the order of our life is never entirely of our own making. Rather, our lives are structured to a great extent by what happens to us, most of which we cannot control. Similarly, the call to be a doctor depends on many circumstances beyond one's control. Many people around the world would make terrific physicians but never have the opportunity to even consider that possibility. Many others, despite ability and interest, will never be offered a spot in a medical school. Such persons, upon realizing that an opportunity to become a physician will not open up for them, must acknowledge that they are not called to the work. They must then think creatively and act energetically to discern a new course—one that may or may not intersect with the world of medicine.

Finally there is need. As is perhaps obvious with respect to medicine, our vocational commitments should respond to needs that we can meet. A life of pursuing human goods is not a self-serving life but a life of self-giving. Here again, we find helpful confirmation in the reflections of some religious traditions. Consider, for example, this claim of the Second Vatican Council: "It follows, then, that if human beings are the only creatures on earth that God has wanted for their own sake, they can fully discover their true selves only in sincere self-giving."[15] In discerning vocation, a person must give special attention to the question of what needs he can address through his ability, opportunity, and interest.

The domain of vocation illustrates a claim we made earlier in this chapter. Although our natural law approach to understanding the requirements of practical reason asserts moral absolutes, it does not assert a one-size-fits-all picture of the moral life. Vocations are personal, requiring that an individual discern both that to which she is called and also that which is therefore required of her (and no longer required of her) in terms of her vocation.[16] The need for such discernment highlights the importance of autonomy in the moral life, including the moral lives of patients and physicians.

CONCLUSION

In chapter 1 we began to articulate the Way of Medicine's understanding of the practice of medicine. In this chapter we have supplemented that inquiry with reflection on the broader requirements of practical reason, which arise from recognizing basic human goods that give us reasons to act for the sake of human flourishing. Recognizing the nature of those goods has led, in turn, to the articulation of three requirements of practical reason: (1) basic goods should never be intentionally damaged or destroyed, (2) we should be fair in our distribution of benefits and burdens as regards other persons, and (3) we should organize our lives around vocational commitments. How does all of this bear on the clinical encounter and the doctor-patient relationship? We now turn to that question.

CHAPTER THREE

The Doctor-Patient Relationship

Let's return to the patients we introduced you to in chapter 1, presenting a bit more information about their specific health concerns:

Cindy Parker goes to student health seeking a prescription for contraceptives.

Abe Anderson asks his physician for antibiotics to treat a respiratory infection.

Nora Garcia wonders if she should have a do-not-resuscitate order.

How should a clinician respond in each of these clinical encounters? What norms guide good medical practice? What kind of relationship should physicians cultivate with their patients, and for what virtues should they strive? The above cases reflect routine encounters between patients and their clinicians, and here in the everyday practice of medicine, we begin to see how the Way of Medicine makes a difference for clinicians in understanding their professional ethical obligations.

Clinicians' approach to their obligations to patients has shifted over the past half-century, contemporaneous with the rise and subsequent evolution of the provider of services model (PSM). Modern bioethics emerged in part because of physicians' abusing their power, both by conducting unethical research on patients and by paying insufficient regard to patients' proper authority to decide how medicine would be deployed on their behalf. In the 1960s and early 1970s, the patients' rights movement contended that traditional medicine gave physicians too much authority, making patients unjustifiably vulnerable to their physicians' whims.

From many quarters came critiques of what came to be called *paternalism* (*pater* is Latin for father), a model of the doctor-patient relationship in which the physician, like a parent, has the authority to tell the patient what to do. The physician orders; the patient obeys. In *strong paternalism*, the good physician would tell Cindy Parker whether to use birth control and which birth control technology to use. He (prior to 1970, almost all physicians were men) would also tell Abe Anderson what to do about his upper respiratory infection and decide whether Nora Garcia would be resuscitated. The physician would make all of these decisions and give the relevant orders based on his superior knowledge of medical science and health. Cindy, Abe, and Nora, as good patients, would obey the physician's orders.

This image of the doctor-patient relationship in bygone days is something of a caricature, of course. Physicians would not stay in business long without cultivating patients' trust and accommodating their concerns. But this image of strong paternalism helpfully marks one end of an ideological spectrum regarding the doctor-patient relationship and the distribution of authority and responsibility within it. It provides a view of what the modern medical ethics movement reacted against: unchecked power, unexamined professional authority, male privilege, and unjustified control over patients.

We do not defend strong paternalism. But we note that shortly after the patients' rights movement successfully established patient autonomy as the driving principle of medical practice, prominent practitioners and critics began to worry that in its retreat from paternalism, the pendulum had swung too far,[1] toward a normative vision of the doctor-patient relationship in which the good patient *chooses* and the good physician *provides*. We see here the essence of the PSM.

The shift from strong physician paternalism to strong patient autonomy depended on and contributed to the growing moral confusion regarding the ends of medicine that Kass described in 1974.[2] That confusion also was described in a seminal 1981 paper written by physician and ethicist Mark Siegler: "Searching for Moral Certainty in Medicine: A Proposal for a New Model of the Doctor-Patient Encounter."[3] As the title suggests, Dr. Siegler was searching for a solid ethical foundation for clinical decisions that doctors and patients would make, and he was doing so at a time in which all such foundations appeared suspect. "What duties, obligations, and responsibilities," he asks, "does the physician incur, voluntarily and autonomously, when he chooses to become a physician?"[4]

Siegler's paper was cited extensively in a 1982 report by the President's Commission for the Study of Ethical Problems in Medicine and Biomedical and Behavioral Research. The Commission wrote:

> The role of the health care professional . . . appears to be in a "phase of incomplete redefinition," . . . "judgments of conscientious persons have become divergent and perplexed" and societal consensus does not exist. No longer are the proper ends and limits of health care commonly understood and broadly accepted; a new concept of health care, characterized by changing expectations and uncertain understanding between patient and practitioner, is evolving. The need to find an appropriate balance of the rights and responsibilities of patients and health care professionals in this time of change has been called "the critical challenge facing medicine in the coming decades.[5]

Almost four decades later, judgments of conscientious persons remain divergent regarding a number of clinical practices, and societal consensus regarding the ends of medicine remains elusive. As we noted with respect to balancing principles, clinicians and ethicists have no way to balance different moral claims without a shared standard regarding the purpose of medicine. What one party (e.g., the patient) judges to be morally and medically necessary, another party (e.g., the physician) may judge to be illicit and unprofessional; benefits and harms depend on perspective. Without a shared standard, then, beneficence defaults to providing what the patient values, and nonmaleficence defaults to refraining from actions the patient does not value.

Justice defaults to requiring the clinician to accommodate the patient's right to choose. As a result, bioethics reduces to a proceduralist approach in which being ethical means determining who has the authority to make a choice and facilitating that choice insofar as possible.

Moreover, the notion of balancing rights and responsibilities suggests that clinicians and patients relate to one another as rivals expecting conflict. The language of balance reflects a focus on defending the rights of one party against those of another rather than on cultivating trust and cooperation around a shared pursuit. In the absence of some objective standard to guide medicine, our culture understandably situates authority with the more vulnerable individual: the patient whose rights are threatened by the physician's power. The responsibility of the physician, then, is not to pursue the patient's health according to the physician's best judgment. Rather, the physician's responsibility is to respect the patient's right to make informed choices regarding which healthcare services the patient will receive, as long as the patient does not request something that breaks the law. By default and prescription, autonomy becomes the overarching principle.

As we noted in the introduction to this book, few physicians consistently follow the PSM. Few physicians would agree, for example, to prescribe antibiotics just because a patient really wants them or to prescribe Adderall for a patient who simply wants to study more effectively. In medical practice, autonomy does not do the work that PSM theory suggests it should. Many physicians implicitly adhere, at least partially, to the Way of Medicine.

We return to our clinical cases to see the difference it makes to understand medicine as the PSM does versus understanding medicine as the Way of Medicine does—as a practice oriented toward the patient's health as one basic human good.

CINDY'S CHOICE

Cindy Parker is a twenty-year-old undergraduate student. She presents to the student health clinic to see a family medicine physician. The physician asks, "What brings you to see me today?" Cindy responds, "I just need a prescription for birth control."

How should the physician in this case respond? Under the PSM, the answer is obvious: prescribe what the patient requests. Why? Because the intervention is lawful and the patient has autonomously requested it. Respect for Ms. Parker's autonomy requires the physician to prescribe the medication unless some unusual condition is present. Moreover, Ms. Parker, like millions of other women, values contraceptives. So prescribing contraceptives satisfies the principle of beneficence—it provides something good for her from her perspective. In addition, contraceptives are relatively safe; they increase the risks of some injuries to a woman's health, such as blood clots in patients who smoke, but such risks remain relatively small and can be mitigated with proper education and triage. Nonmaleficence, therefore, is satisfied. Finally, this is also a matter of justice. Women who take contraceptives are thereby empowered to complete their educational and vocational trajectories and to bear children at times that align with their personal and family needs. It would be arbitrary and unjust for Ms. Parker's physician to refuse to prescribe contraceptives, given that physicians prescribe all kinds of medications that are riskier and achieve goals that patients value much less.

In contrast, the Way of Medicine urges us to ask a different set of questions. The first question is: What do contraceptives have to do with health? In this case, how is prescribing contraceptives consistent with the physician's vocational commitment to preserve and restore the health of Cindy Parker? As we'll see in chapter 6, the answers to these questions are not as straightforward as physicians' customary practices suggest. For the moment, though, suffice it to note that the Way of Medicine suggests it would not be arbitrary for Ms. Parker's physician to decline to prescribe contraceptives if, in the physician's reasoned judgment, the contraceptives either contradict or are beside the point with respect to the patient's health.

ABE'S REQUEST

Abe Anderson is a fifty-year-old carpenter. He has smoked two packs of cigarettes each day for thirty years. Mr. Anderson has a particularly bothersome respiratory infection, with fever, fatigue, and a hacking cough that is productive of thick yellow sputum. His wife has persuaded him to see a physician. Mr. Anderson asks for antibiotics.

This seemingly anodyne case of routine primary care medicine exposes inconsistencies in how physicians understand their obligations, and it opens up critical distinctions between the Way of Medicine and the PSM. Should Abe's physician prescribe the requested antibiotics? If so, why? If not, how can she justify the refusal?

To experienced clinicians it may seem obvious that the physician should judge whether she thinks the respiratory infection is viral rather than bacterial and, if it is viral, she should refuse to prescribe antibiotics. This refusal would be justified because physicians are not obligated to prescribe treatments that do not work (e.g., antibiotics for viral infections), because the principle of justice requires considering the downstream effects of antibiotics on future patients (namely, greater bacterial resistance to antibiotics in the community), and because the principle of nonmaleficence would encourage the physician to avoid the adverse side effects of the antibiotics for Abe, including potential allergic reactions and loose stools. In this case, it might be argued, the physician has strong medical reasons for refusing what the patient requests.

But reality is more complicated. The risk of significant harm to Mr. Anderson from a course of antibiotics is quite low, likely lower than the risk of harm to Ms. Parker posed by long-term use of hormonal contraceptives. Moreover, there is some nonzero probability that Mr. Anderson's physician will mistake the diagnosis, failing to see that Mr. Anderson does in fact have a bacterial infection and would recover more quickly with antibiotic treatment. Doesn't Mr. Anderson have a right to accept the risks of the antibiotics and make an informed choice about whether to take them? Doesn't respect for his autonomy require accommodating his choice?

Apart from the ambiguities posed by probability and uncertainty, we have already noted that the PSM eschews any shared standard against which to judge requirements for beneficence and nonmaleficence. Mr. Anderson might say, "Doc, I value having the antibiotic, even if you do not think it is likely to benefit me. I think it will be good for me, and after all, it is my body and my health we are talking about, right?" He might note that the remote possibility of harm caused by the antibiotics is outweighed by the certain harm of him worrying for days that he might develop bacterial pneumonia, not to mention the cost (another harm) of having to come back to see the physician again if he does.

It turns out that in the PSM, even the claim of having medical reasons to refuse Mr. Anderson's request starts to break down in light of the fact that the profession allows physicians to prescribe antibiotics in such cases, and many physicians do. In the absence of a reasonable standard—say, *health* objectively defined—the physician's medical reasons appear to be arbitrary impositions of power over the patient, unjustly curtailing the patient's right to make informed autonomous choices regarding his medical care.

As both Abe's and Cindy's cases display, invoking midlevel principles does not lead to moral clarity without an account of what medicine is for that might help to specify those principles. Principles can be balanced ad nauseam, but the balancing itself appears arbitrary and determined by power relations unless we presume that medicine is oriented toward a real good that can be known and to which the clinician is reasonably committed.

For the Way of Medicine, Mr. Anderson's case remains complex, but the complexities shift. The physician begins with a commitment to the good of Mr. Anderson's health. Her actions are reasonable insofar as they are conducive to Mr. Anderson's health, and they are unreasonable insofar as they contradict his health. This does not mean that Abe's request has only one ethical response. Medicine is beset by uncertainties and probabilities, after all, and one physician might judge that antibiotics are worth prescribing despite the low probability of benefiting Mr. Anderson's health, because the corollary risk of harm is so low. Another might judge that antibiotics should be avoided despite the low risk of harm because the likelihood of benefiting Mr. Anderson is also low.

According to the Way of Medicine, the physician has the authority to decide which interventions to offer, based on her threshold judgment regarding whether the interventions in question will preserve or restore the patient's health (and there is proportionate reason to accept their side effects; more on that in chapter 5). A good physician will not insist that a patient follow the one route the physician believes is best. The physician may advocate one strategy, but she will allow the patient to choose a different course as long as she determines that the patient-suggested course sufficiently addresses a health-related need and does not violate other moral requirements. Making such determinations is ultimately the work of *clinical judgment*. Physicians attain clinical judgment, which in turn should be guided by the virtue of prudence, only through a combination of experience, reflection, and commitment to the true end of medicine.

NORA'S LIMITS

Nora Garcia is an eighty-year-old widow who in recent years has grown frail. Mrs. Garcia comes for her usual quarterly appointment with her geriatrician. She notes, "I feel like I don't have long to live. I am getting tired. I don't want to be put on all of those machines my husband was put on. Should I have a do-not-resuscitate order?"

What is the doctor's role with respect to Nora? Should he encourage her to make the decision that he believes is best or simply give her the facts? What would characterize good counsel about limiting the use of medical interventions that might otherwise extend Mrs. Garcia's life?

Once again, under the PSM, Mrs. Garcia's physician should seek to help her make the decision that fits what Mrs. Garcia values. The physician should ask her what she cares about and offer her strategies that align with her values, including, perhaps, a do-not-resuscitate order.

The PSM does not encourage the physician to ask what would be a good decision for Mrs. Garcia to make. As long as Mrs. Garcia's choice is permitted by current law and policy, her choosing alone makes the choice ethical. The physician's role is to give accurate information to help her make an informed choice.

By contrast, in the Way of Medicine the physician encounters Mrs. Garcia with a preestablished orientation toward her health. That does not mean that the physician is determined to do everything possible to preserve any measure of health. Indeed, the wise physician acknowledges that health is a good that can be possessed only in part, and only for a time. The wise physician also recognizes that health is not the only good the patient should consider. The physician, then, respects Mrs. Garcia's authority to make judgments about the extent to which efforts to preserve her health fit her vocation, all things considered.

Unlike under the PSM, however, a physician practicing according to the Way of Medicine does not seek a decision that aligns with Mrs. Garcia's *wishes*. Rather, he seeks a decision that makes wise use of medicine (including by putting some limits on medical interventions) to preserve and restore Mrs. Garcia's health, given her vocation and what she will consent to. The physician takes into account the fact that Mrs. Garcia's health is limited, her mortality bears down on her, and other goods might be more important to her than her health. He counsels her to make the decision that, all things considered, he believes is best, and he respects her authority to decline his recommendations. He might readily encourage the patient to have a do-not-resuscitate order. He might encourage her not to. But through it all, he remains committed to serving the health needs of his patient, Mrs. Garcia.

SOLIDARITY AND TRUST

A particular virtue is essential for manifesting and maintaining the commitment to serving patients' health needs: the virtue of solidarity. The relationship between the physician and Mrs. Garcia must be characterized by trust and trustworthiness. In the remainder of this chapter, we address the roles of solidarity and trust in the Way of Medicine.

Solidarity and trust are features of any flourishing community, and also of the community formed between doctor and patient. Recall that physicians' constitutive vocational commitment—the commitment that distinguishes them from philosophers, priests, and dancers—is to health. But physicians do not commit to health in the abstract or even to the health of populations; rather, they commit to the health of *their patients*—that is, health as instantiated in the *particular* persons to whom they attend.

Put another way, a doctor is vocationally committed to a specific kind of community with a particular kind of common good. A *common good* is a good mutually willed by participants in a cooperative, mutually giving relationship. The common good of friends is their friendship, plus whatever other goods they pursue together as friends. The friendship example highlights something that applies universally: one cannot will the common good of a community without also willing the good of the community members. Some group members may be in it for themselves, and if so, they frustrate the possibility of the group's forming a genuine community. Humans can reach their fulfillment only in community, and genuine community, including that formed between a doctor and her patient, requires its members to will and act for each other's good.

Solidarity

Solidarity is the name for this stance without which there can be no common good, no genuine community, and ultimately no human fulfillment. Solidarity is a firm and enduring commitment to the good of other persons and thus to the common goods of one's communities. Solidarity is not simply a concern for the collective, humanity in the abstract, or goods in the abstract. It requires concrete relationships in particular communities, including the relationships that form communities between physicians and patients. The Way of Medicine requires physicians to show solidarity with their individual patients—to be firmly and concretely committed to their patients' good.

But how can a *patient* have solidarity with his doctor, since the purpose of the doctor-patient relationship is to pursue the patient's good? Do doctors and patients not have a rather one-sided community? The answer is simple but important: patients should will the doctor's good in the way that patients can, which is to will their doctor to be a good doctor in all the relevant and necessary ways. The patient wills this not simply so that she will be cured (she might not be, even with the best doctoring) but also because being a good doctor is good for the doctor; through practicing good medicine the doctor flourishes and finds fulfillment as a person. Thus, when a patient treats the doctor as a functionary or lies to or seeks to manipulate the doctor, the patient fails to show solidarity. Such failures of solidarity rupture the community of the doctor-patient relationship as much as do failures of solidarity on the part of the physician.

Physicians can and do fail in solidarity toward their patients. Some doctors are in medicine for themselves, regularly putting a patient's good behind other concerns, such as financial gain, time at the golf course, or the demands of an insurance company. These failures are obvious, but physicians are also prone to two less obvious failures of solidarity.

(1) Physicians can be concerned with medicine and health without being concerned for their patients. Perhaps a physician sees health as a goal and treats his patients as opportunities to achieve health. This detached approach makes some methodological sense. In the surgical operating room, efficiency and effectiveness are often served by treating the patient as an object subject to scientific investigation and technical control. The problem emerges when such treatment is not governed by an overarching commitment to this patient's good. Such patients often report that they were treated "like an object." Insofar as a surgeon sees a patient as a technical problem, for example, he fails to see that patient as a person. Medical subspecialization exacerbates this tendency, habituating physicians to focus only on the diseased or defective parts of a patient rather than on the patient as a whole. Patients also often report that they were treated "like a number," reflecting a tendency for physicians to service as many bodies as possible in the allotted time, often in order to maximize efficiency and profit. Physicians with each of these tendencies, while overtly pursuing health, fail to show the solidarity physicians owe to their patients.[6]

Perhaps a physician is concerned with his professional integrity, but that concern is detached from an orientation toward the good of the patient's health. The doctor may be drawn to an ascetic, unsullied lifestyle as a physician who practices with professional integrity and purity, but his desire to remain above the fray also leads him to detach from human concern for his patients. This condition may seem unusual, but describing it makes the point that a physician's concern for his integrity can become self-centered if that concern is divorced from the patient's health as the end of medicine and if it is not accompanied by the virtue of solidarity. Further, it isn't adequate for a physician to participate only in the community of physicians; in such cases a doctor's allegiance to the guild becomes primary. Allegiance to one's guild can be important, but such allegiance contradicts itself when it displaces the solidarity with patients to which the guild professes and on which the guild's practice depends.

(2) The second failing of physicians is that which most characterizes the PSM: being concerned for the patient's good while denying the possibility of knowing what that good is and what concern for it requires. Such concern reduces to providing patients with what they desire and autonomously choose. In such an approach, there can be no solidarity, for no actual common good exists between the physician and the patient. In practice, many—perhaps even most—physicians and patients break through the constraints of the PSM to form genuine communities with one another, but in doing so they run against and expose the inadequacies of the PSM's logic. Ideas have consequences: if there is no genuine good, there is no good in common; if patients and physicians have no good in common, no genuine solidarity and community are created between them. The logic of the PSM undermines the doctor-patient relationship.

This portrait of the doctor-patient relationship as a community, however, raises a different worry: that the portrait fails to respect boundaries appropriate to the kind of relationship that physicians and patients share. Yes, physicians are concerned for and have solidarity with their patients as whole persons, not as objects or as collections of parts, but surely the whole person includes much that is not the doctor's concern and perhaps none of the doctor's business. Indeed, on the Way of Medicine, the physician's concern is the patient's health, not the entire array of goods that have a place in the patient's life.

We think a middle path exists between the detached posture that treats the patient as an object with whom the physician has no solidarity and the enmeshed mode that, in service to being *holistic*, makes it the physician's business to care about everything that matters to the patient. Patients are living bodily beings, and so the physician who attends to a patient's health—a characteristic of the body as a whole—thereby attends to the patient as a person, even if the physician focuses only on this one dimension of the patient's personal existence. The same is true in other social contexts. Teachers' concern for their students, for example, does not typically extend to the students' home lives, but good teachers nonetheless are concerned for the good of their students as persons. (Think of how odd it would be for a teacher to simply want there to be more knowledge in the world, and to think of students as the objects in which this knowledge was to be realized.) The challenge for physicians and for teachers is to be concerned in the right way.

The right way displays the hallmarks of solidarity. Think, for example, about the importance of listening and communicating in relations between persons. Think also of the virtues that go with listening and communicating well: honesty, tact, patience, and silence, as well as politeness, respect, and humility. These virtues all manifest solidarity: goodwill toward another as a person for whom one has a special care and concern. Such solidarity also requires acknowledging and respecting the patient's authority. The doctor is concerned for the whole person but not by seeking to influence all aspects of the person's life. Rather, respecting the patient's authority, the physician enables the patient to make decisions in the domain of health that fit the patient's vocation as a whole person.

Because the physician ultimately cares for the patient, occasionally that care cannot be confined merely to the good of health (a parallel statement can be made regarding teachers and the good of knowledge). Sometimes physicians can reasonably meet a patient's request for prayer, marital advice, or urgent assistance in some other domain. Physicians need prudence in discerning when such actions complement the physician's vocational purpose—seeking the patient's health—and when they might interfere with or problematically distract from that purpose. The PSM, interestingly, has no way of distinguishing between and ordering the two kinds of actions because it does not distinguish actions oriented toward health from actions oriented toward other aspects of patient well-being.[7]

Trust

Classically the professions respond to particular vulnerabilities that individuals face; such vulnerabilities call for trust on the part of the vulnerable and trustworthiness on the part of those caring for them. Solidarity is so important for the practice of medicine because in order for physicians to help patients, patients and physicians must be able to trust each other.

Patients often seemingly have no choice but to rely on their physicians. Patients do not control when and how they come under their physicians' care, and often they lack the knowledge or wherewithal to evaluate whether the physician is doing a good job. But trust and reliance are different. We rely on something when we simply count on it, and sometimes we count on something when we have no other choice in the matter. Moreover, reliance does not require a personal relationship: you probably rely on your car, but you don't trust it. You don't feel betrayed when it conks out, although you might feel other unpleasant emotions.

Trust, by contrast, entails having faith in some*one*, having confidence that the person will act toward you in ways governed by genuine concern. Children trust their parents once they become old enough to understand the nature of their parents' relationship to them. When older children merely rely on their parents—as providers of food, clothes, and shelter—that evidences a breakdown in the child-parent relationship. Patients certainly rely on doctors—on their technical skills, their showing up during clinic hours, and their billing tools. Yet doctors can prove reliable in all of these and other respects without ever caring about their patients as persons. Such doctors cannot be called trustworthy, as they have no genuine community with their patients. Absence of trust undermines the doctor-patient relationship. The practice of medicine requires a relationship of solidarity, at least according to the Way of Medicine.

CHAPTER FOUR

Autonomy and Authority

In our effort to identify a more adequate framework for medicine, we return to the crucial concept of autonomy. The provider of services model (PSM), in its opposition to the overly paternalistic bioethics of the first half of the twentieth century, has made autonomy its cornerstone concept, overemphasizing it, we believe, to a detrimental degree. That being said, the Way of Medicine also values autonomy, properly understood. In the present chapter, we aim to clarify what good autonomy is and how it relates to the practice of medicine. We also introduce another concept, *authority*, that is essential to understanding the Way of Medicine.

AUTONOMY

Medical practice is shaped by the philosophies of the age. If nothing else, the philosophies of our age emphasize the importance of individuals' directing their own authentic self-expression and self-development. This cultural emphasis has profoundly shaped public expectations of medicine, making autonomy the central feature of contemporary medical ethics. Unfortunately, medical practitioners have come to misunderstand autonomy along the way, and medical ethicists have come to overstate its importance greatly, leading to distortions in contemporary medicine and medical ethics.

Contemporary medical ethics came to focus on autonomy in response to what were obviously violations of autonomy, particularly cases in which medical researchers and practitioners withheld or subjected patients to interventions without the patients' consent. The Tuskegee syphilis experiments are among the most infamous of such cases. Apart from infamous cases, however, physicians often failed to adequately inform patients about their conditions and the courses of action available to them. Physicians also failed at times to obtain consent from patients before enacting the treatment that the physician deemed best. This pattern came to be described as *medical paternalism*, by which physicians assume they know what is best for patients and presume that they have the obligation or right to act for that presumed best. As the Tuskegee experiments show, assuming physicians' benevolence leaves patients unprotected when medical researchers are more interested in societal benefits than in benefits to individual patients. Even when physicians genuinely care about their patients, something important is missing if the patient does not have the opportunity to understand and at least implicitly consent to the physician-proposed treatment.

A move toward autonomy-based medical ethics sought to correct the errors of medical paternalism, but it also dovetailed with intellectual currents that date back to the origins of contemporary liberalism. These intellectual currents hold that our social and political life should recognize and foster people's freedom, equality, and independence. How, people reasonably asked, are freedom and independence upheld when researchers or physicians act on patients without their knowledge or consent? Where is the equality between patient and doctor when the doctor can decide on a course of action unilaterally? Drawing on classical liberal sources such as Immanuel Kant and John Stuart Mill, twentieth-century ethicists argued that the virtues of liberal society could be realized in medicine only through the practice of obtaining informed consent whenever a physician or researcher proposed to do something with, to, or on a patient.[1]

Misunderstandings about Autonomy

Twentieth-century ethicists understandably emphasized informed consent, but on the heels of this emphasis two misunderstandings regarding autonomy have come to distort medical practice.

Misunderstanding 1: An autonomous choice is a right choice. In one view, autonomy is singularly important because what makes a choice right is the autonomy itself. We call this the *radical autonomy* view. By "radical" we do not mean that its advocates operate outside the political mainstream; rather, we mean that in this view the exercise of autonomy itself fundamentally (radical means "at root") affects the nature of the choice, making the choice right.

The radical autonomy view has its origins in the work of Immanuel Kant, for whom autonomy was present only in a choice made in accordance with the categorical imperative: *act only according to that maxim whereby you can at the same time will that it should become a universal law.*[2] A will acting in accordance with such a maxim, argued Kant, was not determined by any incentive such as might be provided by a mere desire; that will was, accordingly, free and autonomous.[3]

More recently, the idea that an autonomous choice is an ethical choice has become detached from the categorical imperative and transformed into something that Kant would not recognize but that some thinkers have dubbed "expressive individualism."[4] According to expressive individualism, the rightness of a choice is a function of its *authenticity*,[5] a conceptual cousin of autonomy. One is authentic if one is one's own person—that is, self-governing and autonomous. A famous expression of this view is found in Supreme Court Justice Anthony Kennedy's decision in *Planned Parenthood v. Casey*, a case involving abortion rights. Kennedy wrote, "At the heart of liberty is the right to define one's own concept of existence, of meaning, of the universe, and of the mystery of human life."[6]

In Kantian ethical theory, respect for another person's autonomy can lead directly to an obligation to obtain that person's consent before engaging in any medical intervention. But as cultural assumptions about autonomy have drifted further from Kant, the view that respect for autonomy requires obtaining informed consent has been supplanted by the view that we owe positive respect to any way in which others "define [their] own concept of existence, of meaning, of the universe, and of the mystery of human life." Stephen Darwall has called this sort of respect "appraisal respect."[7] In the domain of medicine, the radical autonomy view expects medical practitioners not merely to tolerate autonomous choices with which they may disagree; increasingly, this view expects physicians to honor and facilitate such choices.

This expectation of radical autonomy, and the underlying influence of expressive individualism, pop up around many of medicine's most vexing issues. For example, in the realm of death and dying, much of our culture, including important parts of our medical culture, has moved from requiring physicians to respect a dying patient's refusal of further life-sustaining interventions to the view that the dying patient has a positive right to a physician's assistance in dying. Brittany Maynard put it plainly in her online manifesto: "I want to die on my own terms. . . . My question is: Who has the right to tell me that I don't deserve this choice?"[8] Following Ms. Maynard's view, undergirded implicitly by expressive individualism, doctors who care for patients like her must provide death, or the means to death, if that is what the patient autonomously chooses.

For a second example, consider the emphasis on choice that pervades discussions of abortion, contraception, and reproductive questions more generally. As with dying, those who invoke the importance of autonomy increasingly claim not merely that practitioners must abstain from interfering with patients' choices in reproductive matters but also that practitioners must positively respect those choices and help patients carry them out. In this way, medical practitioners' objections to providing abortion or contraception are overruled in favor of what a person has autonomously chosen.

To take up a final issue receiving attention currently, consider the growing movement for transgender rights and equality. We hold that all human persons are equal and equally deserving of basic human rights, whether they are trans- or cisgendered. But many in the transgender movement also hold that an individual's autonomous desire to change gender should be normative for the medical profession. In some states practitioners are legally prohibited from counseling practices that seek to help adolescents sustain a gender identity that matches their biological sex.[9] Medical practitioners are increasingly expected to support and assist those wishing to have their secondary sex characteristics changed through medical and surgical interventions. We discuss the medicalization of gender identity and expression at length in chapter 6.

In these areas and others, the radical autonomy view expects patient autonomy to set the template for what physicians and other medical professionals may, must, and must not do. This misconstrual of autonomy and what it requires, however, undermines the practice of medicine and proves inherently unstable. First, the radical autonomy view reduces the medical practitioner to a kind of functionary whose job is to provide desired services to the patient, regardless of the practitioner's considered judgment about the wisdom or morality of doing so. What matters is patient choice, the central concern of the provider of services model (PSM). This reduction contradicts the Way of Medicine's understanding of medicine as a profession in which practitioners are characterized both by a commitment to the good of health for the patient and by a practical wisdom or clinical expertise related to that good. Under the PSM, practitioners are distinguished not by their wisdom but by technical skills that allow them to accomplish what few others can, and perhaps also by participation in a social contract according to which they may exercise those skills on others if in service to these others' authentic wishes. Lost here is any sense of the physician's calling to serve persons by seeking an authentic and objective good for them.

The radical autonomy view similarly reduces the doctor-patient relationship. In the Way of Medicine, doctor and patient work together to understand, pursue, and achieve what is genuinely good for the patient. Their relationship forms a community of solidarity and trust. The doctor serves the patient, but not in a way disjoined from her own good; indeed, in pursuing the patient's good, the doctor achieves her own good as a doctor. In contrast, if the physician must be in thrall to the patient's desires and choices even when those choices contradict the physician's best judgment, the physician loses the basis for thinking that the practice of medicine coheres with a good life, and the patient loses the basis for trusting the physician to act only for the patient's good.

Moreover, the radical autonomy view proves inherently unstable, for in granting radical autonomy rights to patients, the view unjustifiably eliminates physicians' autonomy. Consider the physician who conscientiously objects to participating in assisted suicide, believing that the practice contradicts the physician's profession to heal and never to harm. In the face of a patient's autonomous demand, the radical autonomy view expects the physician to set her convictions aside or leave the medical profession altogether.[10] But how does this expectation respect the autonomy of the physician? What warrants such an incursion on the physician's capacity for self-government? The radical autonomy position has no good answer.

Misunderstanding 2: Autonomy is the greatest human good. Aside from the claim that an autonomous choice by its nature is a correct choice, a related but different view treats autonomy as the greatest of the human goods—the one that is singularly important for making our lives go well. We call this the *autonomy-first* view.

Those who emphasize autonomy recognize correctly that autonomy and human flourishing are connected, but the autonomy-first view misunderstands the connection. Unlike goods such as health, knowledge, friendship, or religion, which in themselves make a person better off, autonomy makes a person better off only insofar as it is directed toward instances of these and other basic goods.[11] Put differently, an autonomous choice is a good choice only when it is a choice for a good; this can be seen whenever someone makes a self-destructive choice.

Indeed, even a choice for a good can go wrong if the choice is not guided fully by reason. For example, a person who pursues her own health (a genuine good) but does so in a way that disregards foreseeable downstream effects on others (thereby failing to be fair to those others) not only makes a bad choice but also contradicts her own good insofar as her flourishing depends on acting with integrity.

The Importance of Autonomy

Still, autonomy is important to a good and upright life. In the most intuitive sense, autonomy involves a person's freedom to be *self-governing*. This intuitive understanding reflects the etymology of the word: *nomos* is Greek for "law," and *auto* means "self." So an autonomous person is in some way a law unto himself, or self-governing.

But why should people care about being self-governing—deciding for themselves how to live and act? Recall that a good life is lived in pursuit of basic goods, individually and socially. Moreover, a good life is shaped by concern for that life as a whole. We suggested understanding this concern in the sense of a rational life plan, and even more adequately in the sense of vocation: a life of pursuing basic goods for human persons to which one is called and in which one makes good use of one's talents, interests, sympathies, and opportunities.

Such a life clearly requires commitments to goods as well as persons, for at least two reasons. First, some goods—such as friendship, marriage, and religion—are fully realized only by persons who have made commitments, such as to a friend, a spouse, or God. Moreover, these commitments are real only if they are a person's *own* commitments, if she has really made them for herself. This insight, central to arguments for religious liberty, brings into view an initial reason for the importance of autonomy: some human goods cannot be realized at all unless individuals are free to make and follow through on their own commitments.

A flourishing life requires commitments for a second reason that bears even on those goods that can be realized without commitment. Consider, for example, the good of human life. Every baby participates in this good despite not yet making any commitments. But many babies could not enjoy this good were it not for commitments many other people make: doctors and nurses to care for them, researchers who discover new ways of maintaining and fostering human life under adverse circumstances, and family members on whose love and concern the babies depend from the outset of their existence. Commitments help human beings in community realize goods to a greater degree, in themselves and one another.

Such commitments are often social: researchers in any field collaborate and engage with predecessors and successors in pursuing the knowledge they seek. They inherit a body of knowledge and skill with which to work, and they pass new and improved knowledge and skill to future generations. The Way of Medicine itself has built up over centuries through this kind of collaboration.

These commitments, in turn, go better if they are the agents' *own* commitments. Imagine a world in which people are chosen to be doctors and have little say in the matter. In such a world, doctors' flourishing would be stunted by their failure to do what *they* are called to do, and patients would suffer insofar as their physicians fail to be intrinsically motivated for and invested in their work.

Moreover, not everyone is cut out to be a physician, just as not everyone is meant to be a philosopher. Judiciously discerning whether one should commit to one line of work or the other (or both or neither) seems to require taking honest account of one's abilities, dispositions, and opportunities. And who is best situated to take all of these into account if not the person himself, the one who must eventually make the commitment? Again, we need autonomy to deliberate practically about what commitments we should make.

What is true in making commitments is mirrored in their upshot: the obligations that commitments generate. Marital commitments bring marital obligations. The commitment to practice surgery brings obligations for the surgeon. An individual who is best situated to know to what she has committed is likewise best situated to know what obligations follow from that commitment. Individuals aren't free, of course, to make up the obligations that follow from their commitments. A married person cannot reasonably say, "Well, for me, the marriage commitment includes openness to other sexual partners." A surgeon cannot reasonably say, "Well, for me, a commitment to surgery means I get to recommend the surgery for which I get paid the most." Our argument does imply, however, that married persons and surgeons both need the space to make judgments about what their vocational commitments require. Does my marriage commitment mean quitting the job I enjoy so that my wife can pursue the job for which she seems particularly well suited? Does my commitment to surgery mean operating on a patient who is dying even though the odds of success are small? Giving people the space to engage in such discernment and to act on their judgments seems reasonable—more reasonable than deciding for another person what she must do.

For all of these reasons, autonomy, properly understood, contributes a great deal to human flourishing,[12] and physicians go astray if they treat it as unimportant.

AUTHORITY

By deploying the concept of *authority*, practitioners and ethicists can affirm what is true and important about autonomy while avoiding the false implications of the radical autonomy and autonomy-first views.

Medical decisions are made in a social space that includes multiple parties: the patient, the patient's family and friends, the medical professionals involved, and others, such as institutional decision-makers, insurance providers, and clergy. All decisions involving more than one party have a similar problem: given that the various persons involved have different reasons for acting, how do they reach a final decision?

John Finnis has pointed out that there are only two possible ways: unanimity or authority.[13] No further options are available, for unless there is unanimity, every way of making a decision involves some form of authority. Even a vote in which the majority wins substitutes the authority of the majority for the decision of all.

At least two different forms of authority at work in the medical context must be distinguished in order to respect their nature and limits. The doctor typically has the *authority of expertise*. She knows what health is and what interventions will preserve or restore health, as well as in what ways and with what costs and side effects. She also may have the authority of expertise with regard to what the healthiest outcome would be. Sometimes there is clearly such an outcome, and the doctor will speak authoritatively about that outcome to the patient.

But the authority of expertise has its limits. The physician must recognize that the best health outcome (the one most congruent with the patient's medical best interests) is not always the best outcome overall and that often no best health outcome exists anyway. This second, more limited claim implies the first, so let's consider it up front.

In his essay "Searching for Moral Certainty in Medicine," Mark Siegler writes of a professional dancer with asthma.[14] When she begins to seek treatment, the dancer first finds a doctor whose treatment plan allows her to dance but also allows her to suffer some breathing problems, and then a doctor who refuses to offer any treatment plan that does not maximally alleviate her impaired breathing, which requires that she not dance. What seems best to the first doctor—and, importantly, to the patient—is that the dancer be able to dance, even if the treatment that secures that outcome carries risks of impaired breathing. What seems best to the second doctor is that the dancer be able to breathe freely, even though the side effects of effective treatment will leave her no longer able to dance. Is one of these doctors obviously right about the best health outcome? On the contrary: we submit that *no* doctor can say for sure which outcome is the more healthy. Each outcome preserves certain aspects of the dancer's health while leaving other aspects untouched or even impaired.

Moving now to the stronger claim, no doctor can say how important these aspects of health should be relative to the other goods that the patient might seek given her vocation. Being able to dance and being able to breathe seem genuinely incommensurable. So do the risk of death brought on by incompletely controlled asthma and the certainty of not being able to dance brought on by effective asthma medications. The overall outcomes—the health-related outcomes plus the various other benefits and burdens incurred in pursuing those outcomes—are likewise incommensurable. No authority of expertise can discern the best course of action for this dancer in her particular context.

We need a second form of authority. Consider again the claim that even if we focus just on health considerations, sometimes there is no best medical course of action. All medical interventions offer not only benefits but also burdens—side effects that are not chosen but that inevitably accompany the benefits promised. Sometimes, different interventions present very different health benefits, and to pursue one set of benefits often means forgoing the other. In such cases, not achieving one set of benefits is a side effect of seeking to achieve another set. Because the options are incommensurable, the patient may not have the option of choosing a best health-related outcome.

As the dancer's story indicates, health outcomes are not the only ones implicated in medical decisions: medical decisions have consequences for other goods, basic and instrumental. One intervention might keep a patient alive longer but also keep him from fulfilling certain responsibilities. For example, a patient might be offered a special lung transplant that is available only if the patient relocates across the country, away from all family and friends. The patient must factor in such burdens in order to make a wise choice about pursuing the intervention. More generally, an intervention might involve procedures repugnant or immensely painful to the patient, or the intervention might be time-consuming and expensive. In such cases, even where a best possible health outcome seems apparent, the patient still faces a decision about whether, all things considered, pursuing the best health outcome makes sense given the burdens that will follow.

The question is, Who should decide and why? Our answer here plays an important role throughout the rest of this book. The provider of services model (PSM) of medicine, with its singular emphasis on autonomy, sees the answer as straightforward: the patient should decide. The patient should decide either because the right decision is de facto the decision the patient makes (radical autonomy) or because freedom to decide is the most important aspect of human flourishing (autonomy-first). We agree that the patient should decide, but for different reasons. From the perspective of the Way of Medicine, the patient should decide because the patient possesses the *authority* to decide.

Let's step back. Someone or some group must have authority to make that decision. The decision-makers should take into account the various benefits and burdens that follow from different courses of action, but those benefits and burdens are often incommensurable. What standards, then, can be brought to bear to discern a reasonable medical decision?[15] One obvious standard is the patient's health. What can be done that offers a reasonable hope of benefiting the patient's health? The physician, as we suggested above, has the authority of expertise regarding this standard, and therefore the physician has authority with respect to what medical interventions the physician will offer. This genuine form of authority should not be abused or disrespected—not by the physician, who might try to extend this authority beyond its reasonable limits, and not by the patient, who might demand from the physician something the physician believes does not offer reasonable hope of benefiting the patient's health. The physician's authority, which derives from his vocational commitments, thus establishes an initial framework for the choices that the patient must make.

But once courses of action that the physician believes reasonably pursue the patient's health are in view, what standard can be brought to bear to discern the best overall option? This standard should be the patient's vocation.

Think again of Siegler's dancer. The dancer clearly has shaped and will continue to shape her life in terms of those basic goods to which she has made vocational commitments. She pursues her art, and the goods of aesthetic experience and work, with devotion and craft. Perhaps, as for many persons, these commitments are ordered and integrated by other commitments, such as marital or religious commitments. All of these vocational commitments provide a framework within which the dancer reasonably considers the various burdens and benefits her physician offers, and these burdens and benefits together determine what decisions are reasonable for the dancer in this situation.

Note how differently thinking about one's vocation works compared to a bare appeal to autonomy. In the Way of Medicine, the patient can make an apparently autonomous choice and still go wrong. She must be courageous, not allowing unreasonable fear to sway her; she must be prudent, not allowing unreflective desires to lead her away from a reasoned assessment; and she must be just, taking account of her responsibilities and the way that different choices will impact her ability to fulfill her obligations. If our dancer has a small child, for example, it might be both unjust and imprudent for her to pursue dance at the cost of a higher risk of dying. Alternatively, if the risk of death is very low even with suboptimal management of her asthma, she might be cowardly to give up her work and art for the sake of reducing a risk that is already so small.

The patient can go wrong in assessing what her vocational commitments require, but still she has the best epistemic access to what those commitments are and what they imply for this medical decision. The dancer's personal vocation provides the necessary standard for her to reasonably weigh the various incommensurable benefits and burdens of each option and decide which to pursue.[16] She might need advice from someone else to help her consider her options, but even such advice serves primarily to help her take the measure of her own vocation and its implications for her life.

The concept of authority has another feature that autonomy lacks. It helps medical practitioners discern how to respond when a patient chooses a course of action that the physician believes is foolish or even unethical. As everyone knows, authority is no guarantee of its own wise exercise, yet lack of wisdom does not vitiate legitimate authority. Sometimes physicians have good reasons to follow the courses of action that patients choose, even when the physicians are convinced that their patients should have made better choices.

In such cases a physician might reason with a patient and attempt to persuade him that he is exercising his authority in a less than fully reasonable way. Quill and Brody, in a critique of the PSM's tendency to set physicians at odds with their patients, argue that such efforts by physicians to counsel and persuade patients, rather than violating autonomy, actually support "enhanced autonomy."[17] Such efforts do so by giving patients more information to consider in making their decisions. Quill and Brody's critique shines light on deficiencies in autonomy as popularly understood, and we believe their critique would be expressed more adequately in terms of patient authority. After all, if an autonomous choice is self-ratifying, a physician has no reason to argue with or even give more information to someone who has made an autonomous decision. By contrast, prudent exercise of authority often requires consultation with others. Parents have authority over their children, but to exercise that authority wisely they often need to take account of their children's judgments and preferences. Similarly, patients have authority to decide which medical proposals to follow, but to exercise that authority wisely they often need to take account of their physicians' recommendations as well as the input of family and friends and even other healthcare practitioners.

Unlike in the case of autonomy, the concept of authority carries with it limits to that authority. Everyone knows that when political authority is exceeded, the governed have reason to resist illegitimate directives. For example, we commend US Army physicians who have refused to participate in waterboarding and other forms of torture. Their refusals have been justified insofar as orders to participate in torture exceeded the legitimate authority of the ones ordering. Note that we would not commend the same physicians for refusing to obey an order to take care of those prisoners' health needs or even for refusing an order to march into danger with other soldiers, because such orders are within the scope of the legitimate authority of military commanders. Those in power always exceed the scope of their legitimate authority when they pressure the governed to do something that is always and everywhere wrong.

This point about the limits of authority proves important in the medical context. Recall that one complaint against the PSM, with its overemphasis on autonomy, is that it reduces doctors to functionaries who must provide whatever a patient requests. The motto of the PSM is not simply that patients decide (choose), but also that physicians provide (obey). In contrast, focusing on authority makes it clear that sometimes patients will decide, autonomously, that they want something they do not have the authority to demand. This situation arises whenever patients demand that physicians act in ways that contradict physicians' professional commitments.

According to the Way of Medicine, a doctor's professional commitments and expertise give her the authority to decide what she is willing to do within the framework set by her own vocation as a healer. The patient's authority is limited to requesting and then consenting to or rejecting the options made available by the doctor; it does not extend to positive entitlements justified by autonomous choices. Thus, if a patient requests assistance in dying from a physician who, because of moral—including professional—objections, does not offer that option, the patient is well within her authority to seek another physician; but she is well outside the scope of her authority to insist that her doctor provide assistance in dying in the face of the doctor's principled objections.

CONCLUSION

Autonomy matters for human flourishing and to the Way of Medicine. No doubt in the past many physicians claimed a greater scope of authority than was warranted. "The physician decides, the patient obeys" is not an appropriate ethos for the doctor-patient relationship. Respect for autonomy, however, does not mean embracing the radical autonomy and autonomy-first views that undergird the PSM. "The patient chooses, the physician provides" likewise fails as an ethos for the doctor-patient relationship. The Way of Medicine respects the space practitioners and patients need to exercise autonomy, but it recognizes that they have reasonable grounds to do so only within the scope of their proper authority.

CHAPTER FIVE

The Rule of Double Effect

In this chapter we address a final foundational issue before turning to explore the difference the Way of Medicine makes with respect to a number of ethically disputed clinical practices. Our purpose here is to articulate and defend the so-called rule of double effect. This rule plays an essential role in the Way of Medicine. Indeed, as we will show, abandoning the rule of double effect leads directly toward the provider of services model (PSM).

Our framework is robustly pluralistic about basic goods and about the diverse ways that good lives can pursue these many goods. We have argued, however, that some actions are never permissible for anyone. Moral absolutes typically flow from the general norm: basic goods are never to be directly (that is, *intentionally*) damaged or destroyed, whether out of hostility or for the sake of some further good. That norm makes sense, recall, because the basic goods are always good; therefore, hostility toward them is always unreasonable. Basic goods are also incommensurable; it can never be reasonable to destroy one good as a means to achieve a greater good.

The Way of Medicine internalizes this requirement of practical reason, particularly in its understanding of the physician's central vocational norm: never directly (that is, *intentionally*—as end or means) damage or destroy a patient's health and life. This norm starkly distinguishes the Way of Medicine from the PSM, and it has obvious implications where issues such as abortion and euthanasia are concerned, as we discuss in later chapters. But the norm also raises a question: why are moral absolutes, including those of the Way of Medicine, framed in terms of intention?

To explore this question, consider the options that patients typically face: one set of health benefits is linked to one set of health burdens, and another set of health benefits is linked to a different set of health burdens. The options exclude one another. For example, a patient who chooses chemotherapy may have prospects of longer life but will also face significant burdens, including nausea, fatigue, mouth sores, and anemia, all of which diminish the patient's health. Similarly, a patient who declines chemotherapy can expect to avoid these burdens but faces the prospect of dying sooner, a result obviously contrary to the good of life and health. Patients typically cannot avoid making choices that have negative consequences for their health. Insofar as that is true, medicine's chief norm cannot be that physicians must avoid anything that causes damage or destruction to the patient's health. In many situations, physicians cannot possibly comply with such a norm.

Note, however, that in the situation just described, the patient's relationship to the benefits sought or the burdens avoided differs from the patient's relationship to the benefits lost or burdens accepted. A patient who chooses chemotherapy selects a set of health-related benefits and accepts a set of health-related burdens as side effects. Such choices clearly differ from intentionally choosing to damage one's health or choosing to die.

Although a patient cannot always avoid choices that will result in damage to her health, she can, always and everywhere, avoid *choosing to* damage or destroy her health. She can avoid the latter choices even if in no other way than by simply doing nothing. For even if she suffers injury to her health by doing nothing, the injury is, again, a side effect of her (in)action. Thus, moral absolutes speak to what one must never do *intentionally*. This focus on intention is important to *just warfare*—where injury to civilians may be accepted under some circumstances, but never intended. It is also important to the risking of one's life in pursuit of good ends—for example, in fighting forest fires or seeking to rescue someone drowning, and, of course, to the practice of medicine, which inescapably involves accepting the adverse side effects of treatments. Thus, the norm is formulated: never *intend* damage or destruction to a basic good.

ASSESSING SIDE EFFECTS

The rule of double effect can be put quite simply: sometimes an effect that one should never intend can be accepted as a side effect as long as there are *proportionate* reasons for doing so. (More traditional formulations of the rule are more complex; we address them below when discussing intention.)

What is proportionate is one of the most important practical questions in medicine. The answer provides the standard by which to judge many of the most difficult questions physicians and patients face: whether to withdraw or remove treatment when death is not intended but will follow as a consequence, when the death of an unborn child can be accepted as a consequence of actions taken to preserve the mother's life, and many more. Here we provide two general answers to the question about proportionate reason, and we amplify those answers in context in subsequent chapters.

Before saying what a proportionate reason is, however, we should say what it is not. It is not a reason that follows from weighing different goods to find if the "greatest good" will be achieved as a result of the proposed action. If it were possible to take the goods and harms of a proposed clinical intervention and identify which proportion will bring about the greatest good, consequentialism would seem to be a reasonable response. We would want to maximize goods. But if, as we argue, such maximization is not possible, "proportionate reason" cannot refer simply to the balance of good over bad in an option.

Rather, proportionate reason must be understood by considering the goods and harms of an option against a reasonable standard. Two standards are of special importance: fairness and vocation.[1]

Fairness

Recall that emotions and preferences, if not integrated by reason, can distort our choices and blind us to the fact that the basic goods are good for *all* human beings. Thus, a student might lie on his medical school application, knowing that by doing so he is improving his chances of being selected while hurting the chances of other, more highly qualified, applicants. He might think, "I do not know those other applicants, and anyway I need to look out for me." Such thinking, like his act of lying, is manifestly unfair, as the Golden Rule suggests. If six months later we told the student that he did not get into the school of his choice because another student lied on her application, this student would resent the other student's lie.

In this example the effect of one student's lie on another applicant is a side effect. The student does not lie in order to hurt the other's chances of admission. He lies in order to gain admission for himself. He probably recognizes that his action will disadvantage someone else, but that is not his purpose. What makes his action recognizably unfair is that he seeks benefits to which there are burdens attached, and he knowingly takes the benefits entirely for himself while unjustifiably allowing the burdens to fall entirely on someone else. This unfairness is a separate wrong from the wrong of lying.

Similarly, in the case of the Tuskegee experiments, in all likelihood the researchers did not intend the negative effects caused by not treating the subjects in their study. Indeed, they may have rationalized their actions by insisting that, unlike the researchers running some Nazi experiments, they did not directly make their subjects sick. Nevertheless, we can see, and the researchers should have seen, that in not treating their subjects, the researchers sought the benefits of their scientific research and medical knowledge for themselves and others while allowing the attached burdens of the research—sickness and death—to fall entirely on those subjects. The Tuskegee study was therefore manifestly unfair.

Principlists would say that the Tuskegee experiments were failures of justice. Indeed they were, precisely because they were unfair. In general, when principlists and others have drawn attention to abuses of vulnerable populations as subjects of human research, they have pointed out that it is manifestly unfair (and therefore unjust) to take advantage of such populations in order to pursue benefits that those subjects likely will never see while imposing burdens that the eventual beneficiaries will never experience.

Fairness thus provides one standard for judging whether there is a proportionate reason to accept negative side effects. The benefits of an action might be quite significant and the burdens relatively minor, but the action may still fail the test of proportionality precisely because the benefits are distributed to one person or group and the burdens to another. Such an action is unfair unless the person or group receiving all or most of the burdens consents to do so, perhaps out of charity for others whom they wish to benefit, as we see in the case of living organ donors.

As the Tuskegee case illustrates, the standard of fairness in accepting side effects is especially important for the ethical conduct of human subjects research. (Although this book does not focus on it, the norms of the Way of Medicine clearly bear on human subjects research.) Fairness is important for the ethical practice of clinical medicine as well. Physicians can unfairly benefit some patients at the expense of others, can unfairly seek resources for their patients at the expense of their colleagues' patients, or can unfairly privilege their own good over their patients' good. Physicians who begrudge the time they give to a patient because of prejudice, distaste, or dislike for the patient are being unfair, even if they intend no harm.

Fairness does not prohibit physicians from privileging their patients in certain ways. Physicians' commitments to their patients release them from some obligations toward others. In attending to their particular patients, physicians do not attend to those who are not their patients. Indeed, medical practitioners could genuinely care for patients only by privileging their patients in this way. Therefore, this kind of privileging seems to meet the standard of fairness even if, at a given moment, someone is being disadvantaged by it—for example, when a physician sees regularly scheduled patients before patients who arrive without appointments. This kind of privileging seems consistent with the Golden Rule.

Vocation

As we have seen, individuals have good reasons to bring order into their lives by making commitments that orient them toward some goods rather than others. Because human goods are typically sought and obtained in cooperation with other persons, an individual must make commitments to particular persons. Because the goods cannot be sought all at once or all in the same measure, the individual must give priority to some commitments over others.[2]

The individual's vocation names the overall shape of his life—the order brought about by his most important commitments. As we have seen, vocations also generate obligations that require further action. So, for example, a person whose vocation includes a marriage commitment will typically eventually have children, and when that happens his vocational obligations expand to encompass care and concern not just for his spouse but for his children also.

We have made use of this account of vocation to argue for patient authority in healthcare decision-making. Patients have the authority to accept or refuse proposed interventions because they are in the best position to judge whether the benefits and burdens being offered to them are proportionate for them in light of their particular vocational commitments. The patient's vocation provides the standard against which proportionality is judged.

We can see how vocation bears as much on our assessment of side effects as it does on our assessment of what is chosen. Patients make healthcare decisions with benefits and burdens in view, and typically the consequences of their decisions ramify beyond the scope of health. On the one hand, a patient may choose an intervention in hopes of staying alive to spend more time with his family, but as a consequence of the intervention he may experience discomfort, insomnia, and irritability that make it hard for him to be present to his family, do his work, or pray. On the other hand, the patient may choose to decline treatment to avoid the associated burdens, knowing that, as a consequence, he is likely to cut short the time he has to be with his family or engage in other worthy activities. Either decision results in a range of negative side effects, and the patient must judge whether the negative effects to be accepted are proportionate to the goods to be pursued. Vocation provides the standard for that judgment.

DETERMINING WHAT IS INTENDED AND WHAT IS A SIDE EFFECT

Now we return to an overarching question: on what grounds do we discriminate between what is intended and what is merely a side effect?

All action aims at some good. More precisely, all action aims at some state of affairs in which one expects to realize a good. Consider the request for antibiotics by Abe, whom we met in chapter 3. He did not wish merely to possess antibiotics, nor even merely to ingest them. He aimed at a state of affairs in which, the antibiotics having done their work, his health would be restored. So we may say that Abe had a goal or end in mind, and that he hoped to realize the basic good of health in achieving that goal.

To reach this end, of course, Abe had to avail himself of means to that end. He needed a plan, as is true of most of our pursuits of ends. Abe wanted to be healthy; in order to achieve that, he aimed first to take antibiotics; in order to take antibiotics, he first had to obtain a prescription; in order to obtain a prescription, he first had to see a physician; and so on. Put differently, Abe saw a physician *in order to* receive a prescription, *in order to* obtain antibiotics, *in order to* ingest the antibiotics, *in order to* restore his health. In thinking about Abe and each step in this series of actions, we could describe his thinking and his choosing in terms of his plan or proposal for action.

Abe might have considered other proposals; indeed, his physician encouraged him to do so. In the physician's judgment, antibiotics were not a sound means toward health; rest and a tincture of time would be more conducive to health. But at the end of the day, Abe made a choice, adopting one proposal rather than another. The proposal included the end sought—in his case, that state of affairs in which his respiratory infection was healed—and the means to be pursued toward that end. All of this made up Abe's proposal for action, and so all of it was part of Abe's intention.

In contrast, whatever was not part of this proposal—not, that is, either the end Abe sought or the means he chose to achieve that end—can be described as a side effect; it was not part of Abe's intention. Perhaps Abe knew that antibiotics typically upset his stomach and gave him diarrhea. He was not terribly happy about that fact, but he went about seeking and taking the antibiotics anyway. He foresaw that he would feel queasy and have diarrhea for several days, but neither of these consequences was part of his proposal; neither was intended. Although foreseen (more on that below), an upset stomach and diarrhea were neither his goals nor the means he chose to achieve his goal. Falling outside the scope of his proposal, these bad consequences were side effects only.

Even though they were side effects, Abe still bore responsibility for them. He could have chosen a different plan, such as the one his physician recommended, and avoided these side effects altogether. Insofar as Abe was able to choose between different proposals for action, he was responsible for what he accepted as side effects. This is why it was necessary to identify standards—fairness and vocation—by which Abe and others could judge whether there was a proportionate reason for him to accept a particular set of side effects in a particular situation. If we supposed that Abe would in fact benefit from antibiotics and that the digestive issues would not seriously incapacitate him, from the point of vocation, taking antibiotics seems reasonable. But insofar as Abe's expectation of benefit decreased (e.g., as his physician explained that his infection was probably caused by a virus), and his expectation of burdens increased (e.g., if he learned that he was prone to more problematic forms of antibiotics-associated diarrhea), Abe's reasons for accepting these side effects diminished. If they diminished enough, Abe should not have chosen to take antibiotics, even if his doctor was willing to prescribe them. In addition, the doctor in this case had her own decisions to make and her own judgments about proportionality. The doctor had to judge whether the health benefits to be obtained by writing the prescription were proportionate to the side effects of doing so, and she had to consider whether it was unfair to other patients to contribute to antibiotic resistance in the community while pursuing only minor expected benefits for her patient.

Let's return to the question of what Abe intended and a matter of some controversy among philosophers of human action. We have claimed that Abe's intention encompassed all that was included in his proposal or plan—his end as well as all the means he adopted to bring about that end.[3] This claim is controversial insofar as it identifies what was intended from the agent's perspective or point of view. What did Abe seek to obtain, and what means did he choose to bring that about? Abe could choose only by his own lights, but many thinkers, who agree about the importance of intention and the rule of double effect, think that the agent's perspective is too subjective. Motivated in part by some hard cases, they are inclined to argue that one must take a more objective view and that, in some cases, doing so will lead to different conclusions about what Abe chose and whether he chose rightly.

What hard cases do they have in mind, and how do those cases bear on how we think about intention? The body of writing about intention is enormous, but here we focus on a case famously presented by philosopher Philippa Foot. Foot described a case involving cave explorers trapped by a landslide that had left one of their number blocking the only way out of the cave. Water in the cave was rising fast, and the only way to move the man and the rocks that were pinning him was to use a single stick of dynamite to blow open a hole through which the explorers could escape—all the explorers except, of course, the one who was stuck, whom the explosion would kill.

Would it be homicide to blow open the hole? Would those who blew open the hole necessarily intend the man's death? By our account, as described above, it does not seem that the explorers' proposal included the man's death. Their end was to save their lives. The means they chose included blowing open a hole in order to escape. On our account of their intention, the explorers would not be guilty of intentionally killing the man stuck in the hole. (Whether it would be permissible to accept his death as a side effect is a separate question, which would clearly require a consideration of fairness and vocation.[4])

But many find this conclusion appalling. Surely one cannot blow a hole open by setting off a stick of dynamite right next to a living human being and not intend that person's death! The action of setting off the dynamite and causing the death of the trapped explorer seems, as philosophers say, "too close." Thus, on some theorists' account, if the bad effect is too close to the action, it should be considered part of what is intended, even if the bad effect is not part of the agents' proposal. The challenge in such accounts is not only to distinguish that which is part of a person's proposal from that which is not, but also to discern whether bad effects are sufficiently close to the action to be considered part of what is intended, thus making the action unreasonable.

One of the authors of this book has addressed the problem of closeness at great length elsewhere,[5] and we do not propose to wade further into that topic here. But we mention these different accounts of intention here because they return in chapter 7 when we discuss some disputed questions related to the beginning of life.

Articulating the Rule of Double Effect

We are now in a position to compare our formulation of the rule of double effect with the more common and somewhat more complicated formulations.

Above we presented the rule as follows: sometimes an effect that one should never intend can be accepted as a side effect as long as there are *proportionate* reasons for doing so. This formulation is relatively simple, and it leads to a relatively simple way of applying the rule: only intend (i.e., will or choose) the good, and only accept the bad side effects of an action when there are proportionate reasons for doing so (with proportionality judged against the standards of fairness and vocation).

A more traditional formulation of the rule is somewhat more complicated. According to that formulation, one may accept the bad effects of an action if the following four conditions are met:

1.   The act is good in itself (sometimes stated as *the act is not intrinsically wrong*).
2.   The bad effect is not intended.
3.   The good effect is not achieved by means of the bad effect.
4.   There is proportionate reason for accepting the bad effect.[6]

We prefer our simpler formulation, because we believe it encompasses these four conditions. *Only intend the good* encompasses conditions 1 through 3. An action that intends only the good is good in itself. Because, on our account, one's intention includes both the end one seeks and the means one chooses to bring about that end, conditions 2 and 3 are redundant and can be stated simply as *never intend the bad* (the logical corollary of *only intend the good*). Finally, our formulation includes the requirement of proportionality (condition 4).

RECOGNIZING THE CLINICAL IMPORTANCE OF THE
RULE OF DOUBLE EFFECT

We conclude this chapter by pointing to the pervasive role that the rule of double effect plays in medicine and medical ethics. Physicians lean on the rule of double effect in their everyday reasoning about whether the adverse side effects (the language physicians have long used) of a treatment should be accepted in light of the benefits that the treatment promises. Physicians cannot possibly honor the ancient medical commitment to do no harm except by either doing nothing, and so failing to be physicians, or by deploying the rule of double effect—intending only the good to be brought about by an intervention and accepting the bad side effects only when there is proportionate reason to do so. Physicians thus tacitly deploy the rule of double effect whether or not they explicitly embrace it or the Way of Medicine. Therefore, we might say that those who critique the rule of double effect find themselves critiquing their own everyday clinical practices.

The rule plays a more visible and equally foundational role when we turn from every-day, uncontroversial practices to ethically controversial interventions. Without the rule, one cannot, in many cases, respect all persons by not violating their goods—goods that moral absolutes protect—and still act to preserve and restore the health of one's patients. Application of the rule of double effect is essential, for example, in showing how an intervention to save the life of a pregnant woman need not violate the norm against intentional killing, even when the intervention will result in the death of an unborn human person. The rule is equally essential for understanding the difference between the practices of withholding or withdrawing medical treatment and the practices of assisted suicide and euthanasia.

Finally, the rule of double effect plays a critical role in the question of cooperation, a central question wherever physicians are pressured to act against their conscience. Medical practitioners cooperate in unethical practices whenever they do something that makes it easier for another person to do something bad. For example, suppose a patient asks for a referral to an unscrupulous pain physician because the patient intends to get opioid medications in order to abuse them. If the practitioner intends to make the bad action easier to take—that is, makes the referral so that the patient will be able to abuse opioid medications—the practitioner formally cooperates, and formal cooperation is always unethical; it is always wrong to intend what is bad. But if the practitioner does not intend to make the bad action easier, the physician only *materially* cooperates, and the question then becomes, Is there a proportionate reason to accept the unintended bad as a side effect? So put, the question of cooperation clearly requires application of the rule of double effect.

CONCLUSION

The rule of double effect plays a pervasive and foundational role in the Way of Medicine. The rule undergirds physicians' routine practices of assessing side effects, and it protects them from violating the moral commitments that have guided physicians for centuries in the Way of Medicine. Therefore, we encourage the reader to be wary of those who dismiss the rule because it was first articulated formally in a religious community (Roman Catholic, to be precise) or because intentions are often hard to judge from the vantage point of a third party (they are indeed sometimes hard to judge, but that does not make intentions less important) or because the rule seems to limit the scope of a patient's right to self-determination (it does, which is why medicine requires the concept of authority).[7] The profession of medicine detaches from the rule of double effect to its peril.

CHAPTER SIX

Sexuality and Reproduction

The clinical terrain involving sexuality and reproduction includes an expansive array of ethically controversial topics. With respect to sexuality, these topics range from gender and sex transition to sexual performance to the prevention of pregnancy. With respect to reproduction, they range from genetic counseling and assisted reproductive technologies prior to pregnancy to prenatal genetic diagnosis and abortion during pregnancy to resuscitation of neonates and surgical sterilization after pregnancy.

In no other domain do the provider of services model (PSM) and the Way of Medicine diverge more starkly. According to the Way of Medicine, the constitutive end or purpose of medicine is the patient's health. No one should intentionally damage or destroy basic goods, and health and other goods should be pursued by physicians only in ways that are fair to others and that respect one's vocational commitments. The domain of sexuality and reproduction gives a clear picture of what the practice of medicine looks like when it abandons these principles in favor of elevating patient autonomy, choice, and subjective *well-being*.

To organize our approach to this domain, in this chapter we follow two of our previous cases and add another in order to focus on three prominent topics: contraception, assisted reproduction, and gender and sex transition. In chapter 7 we turn to the issue of abortion.

Before going further, we note a looming difficulty. Clinical ethical controversies regarding sexuality and reproduction disproportionately focus on and have consequences for women. Moreover, the approach we advance, in which medicine is oriented to health as one among several basic human goods, leads to conclusions that many will see as contradicting women's "reproductive rights and freedoms" and women's well-being more broadly conceived. If that were not enough, both of us are men, a fact that to some readers makes us unqualified to address questions that bear more heavily on women. For all of these reasons, we proceed with caution, but we proceed nonetheless.

THE PILL AND THE NEW MEDICINE

Whether the advent and subsequent dissemination of contraceptives should be celebrated or lamented (a topic we address below), "the pill" profoundly altered what patients expect of physicians and what physicians expect of themselves. We noted earlier that as biomedical science has expanded, it has made possible many uses of medical technology that are not obviously directed toward preserving and restoring health. The paradigmatic example of such interventions, and perhaps the most consequential for medical ethics, is the contraceptive.

In 1979, roughly twenty years after the US Food and Drug Administration (FDA) approved the first oral contraceptive,[1] Mark Siegler and Anne Dudley Goldblatt wrote,

> The oral contraceptive medication was the first prescription drug that was (and is) in effect, a self-prescribed "treatment." Patients—i.e., medical consumers desiring elective medication— demanded that physicians prescribe the contraceptive pill. Other popularly self-prescribed medications soon followed . . . [and] came to be seen as appropriate solutions or treatments for problems previously considered individual or social concerns, but in any case not biological abnormalities or specific diseases.[2]

Siegler and Goldblatt, neither of whom had any moral objections to contraceptives as such, nevertheless worried that the widespread prescription of contraceptives by physicians established a problematic pattern in which patients pursue and receive interventions that have biological and physiological consequences—and so are sought from physicians who are licensed under US law to "provide" such interventions—and yet are not clearly required by physicians' traditional orientation to the health of their patients. They worried that this widespread pattern was leading to the phenomenon of the "demanding patient" and was teaching patients and physicians alike to think of the physician as a mere provider of healthcare resources.

Public perceptions and expectations regarding physicians have continued to shift in the directions Siegler and Goldblatt worried they would. As we discuss below, prescribing contraceptives is not obviously congruent with an orientation to the patient's health, yet prescribing contraceptives has come to be seen as obviously part of a physician's task. To support this shift, *health*, objectively defined, has steadily been displaced by a much more expansive notion of *women's health* (a version of *well-being*) that includes sexual and reproductive autonomy and reliable family planning. This shift leads physicians to detach from practicing medicine under the Way of Medicine's orientation to their patients' health in favor of "providing healthcare services" according to the wishes of their patients. In the former, the physicians' judgment is essential. In the latter, that judgment is either irrelevant or an impediment to their patients' achieving well-being.

There is a logical progression to these shifts:

1. People desire a state of affairs (e.g., temporary sterility) that doctors can bring about.
2. The desired state of affairs is not obviously related to health.
3. The aims of medicine, therefore, are broadened, either by adding to health other aims (e.g., reproductive autonomy) or by expanding the definition of health (e.g., to well-being) so that it includes these additional aims.
4. Physicians cannot, as a result, have the authority that comes with expertise regarding the aims of medicine since they have no authority of expertise regarding this expanded set of concerns (e.g., whether and when women should be open to pregnancy).
5. Physicians should be nondirective in their counsel to patients, giving accurate information but letting patients decide how and when their physicians will cooperate to bring about the states of

affairs that the patients desire (whether sterility, pregnancy, or something else altogether).

These shifts in public and professional understandings put pressure on physicians to either go along or leave the profession, and they underpin the swing of the pendulum from paternalistic medicine to the patient-as-client model undergirding the PSM. The pendulum received a decisive push when family planning was incorporated into the domain of medicine.

CONTRACEPTIVES IN THE CLINICAL SETTING

Cindy Parker, the twenty-year-old undergraduate student we met in chapter 1, presents to the student health clinic to see a physician. The physician asks, "What brings you to see me today?" She responds, "I just need a prescription for birth control."

In the context of the PSM, it is hard to see anything ethically interesting about this interaction. Ms. Parker requests contraceptives, as the great majority of American women do at some point in their lives. Indeed, prescribing contraceptives is one of the most common and routine practices of obstetrician-gynecologists, family physicians, and others who care for women of child-bearing age.

The Provider of Services Model

According to the PSM, prescribing the pill to Ms. Parker is uncontroversial, if not ethically obligatory. First, contraceptives meet the criteria of being legal, technically feasible, and readily available in the present context. The physician needs only to write a few words on a prescription pad, something that physicians are eminently competent and qualified to do. Meeting these criteria implies that the intervention (contraception) is among those options that a physician must offer to a patient in order to duly respect the patient's autonomy. The physician might ask Ms. Parker questions and share information with her about the actions and side effects of different contraceptives in order to make sure her request is free and informed, but after doing so the physician must honor Ms. Parker's choice.

Notably, in the principlist framework favored by the PSM, the principle of beneficence also moves the physician to prescribe the contraceptive, insofar as only Ms. Parker is in a position to decide what is good for her—that is, whether a contraceptive will contribute to her well-being or not. Only she is in a position to consider the various states of affairs that she values, such as finishing her degree and advancing in her career, as well as enjoying sexual intimacy when that seems right to her. She may hope to have children one day, but pregnancy now would substantially disrupt her life plan. Contraceptive technology allows her to pursue her goals without the fear of becoming pregnant.

To this basic structure of reasoning, PSM proponents may add other considerations. They may note that contraceptives are relatively safe. Although the PSM is often willing to set aside the health of the patient in order to achieve other patient goals, to date most ethicists have supported physicians who declined to provide interventions that threaten imminent substantial bodily harm to the patient (some exceptions are addressed below). So, for example, surgeons are supported in refusing operations that will cause significant harm and have little prospect of restoring health. Contraceptives, by contrast, do not seem to reach that threshold. Contraception-associated risks of major harms such as blood clots and stroke remain small. Moreover, pregnancy brings its own health-related risks, so that a harms-reduction model appears to support using contraceptives to minimize bad health outcomes downstream.

Then there is the question of justice. Access to effective contraception has made it possible for millions of women like Ms. Parker to pursue vocational pathways that early motherhood might foreclose. As such, many would argue that Ms. Parker has a justice claim that the physician must respect.

Ultimately, only Ms. Parker is in a position to weigh all of the desired and undesired consequences of using or not using contraceptives in order to make an informed choice about whether a contraceptive is right for her. In light of all this, it seems obvious under the PSM that the physician should prescribe what Ms. Parker requests.

The Way of Medicine

On the Way of Medicine, this same case becomes problematic. Our framework starts not with the question of whether prescribing contraceptives is legal, feasible, and available but instead with the question of whether prescribing a contraceptive is congruent with the physician's commitment to her patient's health. The answer to that question is not obvious in this most common of cases, insofar as being capable of pregnancy is a sign of health for a woman of Ms. Parker's age. Prescribing a contraceptive thus fits awkwardly with a commitment to health, if it does not indeed contradict that commitment.

We can imagine cases in which our framework might straightforwardly affirm the prescription of drugs that in most cases are used as contraceptives. For example, hormonal contraceptives are often prescribed to treat medical conditions such as endometriosis or bleeding fibroids, or even to restore healthy menstrual patterns. In such cases, the physician who prescribes the drug seems to do so for the patient's health. Temporary sterility is foreseen as a side effect in such cases, but it need not be and often is not intended, and there is often a proportionate reason to accept the side effect.

In the usual case, however, as in Ms. Parker's, physicians prescribe contraceptives not to preserve and restore health but rather to make the patient temporarily sterile. That action not only departs from the physician's commitment to patient health but also seems to contradict that commitment. Pregnancy is a sign of health for a young woman who engages regularly in sexual intercourse. Indeed, if Ms. Parker were to tell her physician that over the previous three years, she and her boyfriend have had sex regularly without using condoms or other contraceptives, the physician then would have good reason to think that something is wrong with the health of Ms. Parker or her boyfriend. So when a physician directly diminishes a patient's fertility—by prescribing a contraceptive or conducting a sterilization procedure—she thereby directly diminishes her patient's health.

Does this argument define *health* too narrowly? Contraceptives may diminish one dimension of health, but what about the proper working of the organism as a whole? How can the health of Ms. Parker on a contraceptive be considered deficient relative to the health she would have if she were thirty-six weeks pregnant, with swollen legs, elevated heart rate, and a reduced capacity for exercise? Moreover, what about those risks of injuries to health that pregnancy brings: bleeding, infections, a ruptured uterus, even death? These questions have force, particularly when a woman has a condition, such as a congenital heart defect, that puts her at markedly elevated risk of harms to health during pregnancy. Within the framework we propose, it is along such lines—orientation to a patient's health—that a physician should ask himself whether prescribing a contraceptive in a particular case coheres with or contradicts his profession.

In this respect, the case of being called on to prescribe a contraceptive might seem similar to other instances in which a physician seems to engage negatively with one dimension of a patient's health for the sake of others. Thus, amputation of a limb removes a part of the organism for the sake of the whole; surgery involves cutting into healthy tissue to get at the unhealthy. Is the provision of a contraceptive similar to either of these instances?

We think not. Effecting temporary sterility is at least a suppression of a patient's healthy functioning in a way that removal of a gangrenous limb is not. Once a limb or organ is gangrenous, there is no state of health available to the organism except one in which the diseased part is removed. That new state—without the diseased part—is clearly a state of improved health relative to the state in which the diseased part remains intact. A parallel situation occurs when a dying patient is suffering terminal agitated delirium; then "cutting off" the diseased state of consciousness using sedatives may restore the only measure of health available to a person in that condition—one clearly reduced relative to a healthy organism but improved relative to that particular state of agitated delirium. We discuss this further in chapter 9. Intentionally causing temporary sterility in a case like Ms. Parker's differs from these cases. Fertility is not like gangrene or delirium; rather, causing temporary sterility in this case seems to involve reducing the health of the whole for the sake of preserving some dimension of health, or at least being hostile toward one dimension of health (that dimension which makes reproduction possible) for the sake of other dimensions.

Contracepting also differs from accepting the incidental damage to health that inevitably occurs as a side effect of medical interventions. In *Hippocrates' Oath and Asclepius' Snake*, Thomas Cavanaugh notes that these "wounds of treatment" inevitably accompany all medical efforts to restore order to a dis-ordered body, but the wounds are not intended. Indeed, medical progress is measured in part by mitigating the wounds that accompany medical interventions. In the case of contraception, however, the physician intentionally suppresses healthy function as a means to some other goal—even a health-related goal. Doing so seems to contradict the physician's professed and fundamental orientation to health and thus to be an instance of what Cavanaugh calls "role-conflation" harm—harm that is intended by the physician contrary to the demands of her profession.[3]

To summarize, prescribing contraceptives, at least in Ms. Parker's representative case, contradicts the physician's commitment to the patient's health; contracepting is not, to put the point more strongly, *medicine* at all, even if it has many of the trappings of medicine.

This verdict of the Way of Medicine is supported by reflection on the requirements of practical reason. Practical reason converges with the Way of Medicine in an argument against contraception that turns on the way that using a contraceptive seems sometimes to involve hostility toward the child who might otherwise come into existence as the fulfillment of sexual intercourse. We argued in chapter 5 that one intends what one adopts in one's proposal for action, encompassing both the end one is pursuing and the means one chooses to bring about that end. In contraception, one anticipates an action—engaging in sexual intercourse—that could result in a child as a consequence, and one wishes to prevent that consequence. So one chooses a contraceptive as the means to prevent a child's coming into existence. This action seems contrary to the good of human life.

Some thinkers have gone as far as to argue that the choice to contracept is structurally similar to the choice to abort. Contraception and abortion are not the same wrongs, for there is no actual child in the case of contraception, but a culture in which the great majority of people intentionally prevent the existence of innumerable possible children would not surprisingly extend its efforts to prevent children from being born by also supporting the practice of abortion. Indeed, if children are expected to follow from sexual intercourse only when their existence is wanted, abortion becomes a critical backup strategy for dealing with unwanted pregnancy. In the Supreme Court case *Planned Parenthood vs. Casey*, the Court noted, "For two decades of economic and social developments, people have organized intimate relationships and made choices that define their views of themselves and their places in society, in reliance on the availability of abortion in the event that contraception should fail."[4] Contraception turns out to be not so much a bulwark against abortion as a gateway to it.[5] Of course, if abortion is not morally problematic, this suggestion will bring no disquiet. As we will show in chapter 7, however, abortion itself gravely violates the good of human life.

ASSISTED REPRODUCTION

Abe Anderson remarried three years ago. His wife is now forty-three years old and has not gotten pregnant despite their deep hopes to have children. Mr. Anderson and his wife present to her ob/gyn asking for help in achieving pregnancy

The Provider of Services Model

The PSM approach to this clinical moment can be summarized briefly, as prior themes are repeated here. Respect for patient autonomy gives us a reason to do what the Andersons ask. In contrast to Ms. Parker, Ms. Anderson wants to be pregnant, so the state of pregnancy is good *for her*; beneficence compels clinicians to pursue that goal. The law, particularly in the United States, where regulations are few, permits quite a range of technological interventions to bring about pregnancy, and many physicians make those interventions available; physicians are also compelled by what is customary and standard. Moreover, most assisted reproductive technologies involve pharmaceuticals or surgical interventions that only physicians are licensed to provide, so Ms. Anderson seems to have a justice claim—that her physician should make available that which is legal, which others readily obtain, and to which she has access only with a physician's help.

The principle of nonmaleficence seems to countervail these imperatives to some extent, insofar as many assisted reproductive technologies pose risks to the woman's health. For example, in vitro fertilization (IVF) involves the risks posed by ovarian hyperstimulation and surgical retrieval of oocytes. As noted above, the state of pregnancy itself brings risks to health that tend to increase with age. But unless these risks reach the threshold of directly and imminently causing major bodily injury, physicians must defer to their patients to weigh the risks and benefits, broadly construed, and make the choice that is best for each individual patient—that is, the choice that maximizes all of the goods, as she defines them, available to her.

Curiously, in the domain of sexual and reproductive healthcare, the PSM leads us to treat the same state of affairs as good and to be sought for one patient and as bad and to be avoided for another patient; the only difference is whether the patient wants the state of affairs. Unlike the Way of Medicine, which focuses consistently on objective human goods, the PSM detaches from the question of whether a possible state of affairs brings about genuine good, considering only whether that state of affairs is wanted.

The Way of Medicine

Assisted reproduction becomes problematic on the Way of Medicine. The physician again asks, in the first instance, what accommodating the Andersons' request has to do with her commitment to preserve and restore Ms. Anderson's health, but here the answer is a bit more complicated. If Ms. Parker had regular sexual intercourse without contraceptive measures from ages eighteen to twenty-one and did not become pregnant, that would be evidence of something wrong with her health or the health of the man with whom she had regular intercourse. Is the same not true for Ms. Anderson?

Yes, it is, although Ms. Anderson's case highlights that health is always relative to a person's sex and age. To state the obvious, no physician to our knowledge would consider it a medical problem that *Mr.*

Anderson has not achieved pregnancy, because the health of men does not include child-bearing capacity. Similarly, physicians would not at this time consider it a medical problem that Ms. Anderson had not achieved pregnancy if Ms. Anderson were eighty years old. The health of eighty-year-old women simply does not include the capacity to bear children. Ms. Anderson, forty-three years old and premenopausal, is at a point in life in which the capacity for pregnancy is characteristically diminished relative to, say, that of a twenty-three-year-old woman, but some healthy forty-three-year-old women do become pregnant. Therefore, in the Way of Medicine, the fact that Ms. Anderson has not become pregnant does give the physician a reason to get involved—but in what manner, and why?

First, what is the physician's goal in this case? The initial reaction might be, "A baby, of course." After all, the only reason Ms. Anderson wants to be pregnant is that she wants a baby—presumably a baby that is genetically hers and her husband's. If the physician had a reliable way to bring about pregnancies, but such pregnancies would inevitably end in spontaneous abortion, Ms. Anderson would not be interested in the physician's help. Yet we have already said that health is the proper goal of medicine, and a baby is not health, so although the physician might reasonably join the Andersons in hoping that their sexual union will result in a baby's being conceived and born to them, the baby—however good and however strongly desired by the Andersons—lies outside the proper scope of the physician's practice.

To give a parallel example, Ms. Anderson might suffer from minor arthritis that many people would ignore but that keeps her from an activity that she highly values—say, a form of dance to which she has devoted much of her life. In such a case, as the physician attends to her arthritis, the physician might join her in hoping that she will dance again and might readily understand why this condition that others consider trivial concerns her so much. Yet the physician's goal is not dance but the health that makes dance possible. Similarly, the physician's aim with respect to Ms. Anderson's desire to have a child is the health that makes pregnancy and subsequent childbirth possible.

Within the Way of Medicine's approach to Ms. Anderson's health, much can be done. Physicians might seek to restore healthy patterns of ovulation, sometimes through attention to nutrition and exercise and sometimes through pharmacological interventions—including medications typically used as contraceptives—such as exogenous hormones to replace or return to normal levels those that are disrupted in one way or another. Physicians might intervene via hysteroscopy or laparoscopic surgery to restore patency to the woman's fallopian tubes. In parallel, a physician might work to improve any deficiencies in Mr. Anderson's capacity to produce healthy semen, including viable sperm; to achieve and sustain an erection; and to reach ejaculation. All of these interventions might be reasonably carried out on the Way of Medicine. These practices are standard for doctors who focus on responding to infertility, and today a minority of such physicians explicitly limit themselves to such practices. The latter include those who put themselves forward as practitioners of NaPro Technology (natural procreative technology).[6] These physicians aim at health, hoping that such health will be followed by pregnancy and childbirth, much as physicians treating arthritis aim at health, hoping that such health will enable dancing and other activities that display health.

As we have noted, the PSM is willing to circumvent health altogether in order to produce a baby. Indeed, this willingness characterizes the entire terrain of contemporary reproductive medicine in the United States, rightly characterized by many as a kind of Wild West in which all things are permitted. Physicians practicing in this area engage in artificial insemination, in vitro fertilization, surrogacy, and other interventions intended not to restore or preserve health but instead to use technology and the remaining health-related capacities available to bring about the birth of a wanted baby.

PSM-focused physicians will readily subject a woman to substantial risks to her health if she is willing to undergo such risks in order to conceive a baby. Gonadal hyperstimulation, for example, is known to cause ovarian hyperstimulation syndrome, which brings an array of health problems and in severe cases can be life-threatening.[7] In the case of oocyte donors, physicians subject the women to these risks while also treating them instrumentally, as means to satisfy someone else's desires. In gestational surrogacy, physicians likewise treat the surrogate mothers as instruments to satisfy another's desires while they impose on the gestating woman all of the risks that accompany pregnancy. The problem is not so much that physicians tolerate side effects but that they tolerate side effects that damage health in order to obtain states of affairs that have nothing to do with the physicians' commitment to this good. For these reasons, simply on the basis of their constitutive commitment to the patients' health, physicians have reasons to avoid many assisted reproductive technologies.

As with contraception, the requirements of practical reason converge with the Way of Medicine's judgments on these types of interventions. Consider the argument against those assisted reproductive technologies that separate procreation from sexual intercourse. In brief, interventions such as IVF seek to *make* a baby, exerting mastery over the raw materials of nature (gametes) by using the technologies available to bring into being a desired product, in this case, a living human being. As with other instances of making, the product comes into existence at the pleasure of the makers, who accept the product on the condition that it satisfies the desires that led them to engage in the productive process. This feature of conditional acceptance is manifested in the widespread practices of grading embryos, discarding suboptimal embryos, selectively reducing embryos when an undesired number have implanted, and cryopreserving, and perhaps donating to science, "spare" embryos.

We develop the argument further in chapter 7, but here we note that human beings at the embryonic stage are still human beings and therefore deserve the basic respect that we accord to other human beings—especially the respect of not being killed. Nor should we treat any human being, including a human embryo, as merely a product or a thing to be brought into existence at will, for doing so radically contradicts the demands of equality that are central to the good of friendship even in its thinnest and most extended sense.

In this sense, human beings are called to a kind of friendship with all other human beings, in virtue of recognizing that all other human beings also are fulfilled by basic human goods. This minimal friendship requires us to treat all human beings with equal respect. Thicker forms of friendship build on this basic form: even when children cannot yet reciprocate, parents act for the good of their children as part of their good as parents. In the full paradigmatic form of friendship, each friend treats the good of the other as his own good.

IVF and related practices undermine the good of friendship by treating another human being as a product—as some*thing* whose existence is subject to one's own will and mastery. These practices undermine friendship even in its thinnest form, for no human being wishes to be treated as a thing by another. Moreover, these practices are deeply at odds with the form of friendship parents characteristically demonstrate toward their children, in which they neither make their children the objects of their will nor make their love contingent on the childrens' satisfying the parents' desires. One who accepts you only on the condition that you satisfy their desires cannot be called your friend. With respect to conjugal intercourse, the attitude appropriate to friendship is fully open to, if not also hopeful for, that act's finding its fullest realization in a new life over which the woman and the man ultimately have little control.

Thus, in vitro fertilization, human cloning (if and when it arrives), and even more limited technologies such as artificial insemination all seem morally impermissible. Once again, we have only sketched the argument, which has been presented elsewhere at greater length and with attention to objections.[8] But our overall aim here has been to show that the Way of Medicine and the requirements of practical reason converge in their conclusion that the Wild West of assisted reproductive technology needs reform. At present, its modes of practice are deeply at odds with the purposes of medicine and the demands of practical reason.

SEX AND GENDER IN TRANSITION

Jules Baker, an otherwise healthy thirteen-year-old boy we haven't introduced you to before, suffers from gender dysphoria. He identifies as female and wishes to take hormone-blocking supplements that will delay puberty until he is old enough to undergo a full sexual transition: sexual reassignment surgery to remove his male sex organs and provide female facsimiles by means of plastic surgery.

The Provider of Services Model

The cases of Ms. Parker and Ms. Anderson make plain that physicians practicing in accordance with the PSM will often set aside the norm of the healthy organism if doing so accommodates the autonomous choices of patients. So, under the PSM, whether the physician works to induce sterility or enhance fertility, to get rid of pregnancy or produce it, often depends entirely on the patient's choice. Physicians respectfully refrain from drawing conclusions about the signs of a "healthy" human organism until they know what a particular human being wants with respect to his or her body.

The case of Jules indicates how far this logic extends in contemporary medicine. If the signs of health with respect to sexual intercourse and pregnancy depend on the wishes of the patient, why not also the signs of health with respect to secondary sex characteristics? If the goals of medicine are rightly determined by the informed choices of autonomous patients—by what patients determine is good for them—perhaps the form of "healthy" secondary sex characteristics should also be determined by the informed choices of patients—by what patients decide are the right secondary sex characteristics for them.

We now see a burgeoning practice of what have come to be called *gender transition* and *gender-affirming* services—the use of exogenous hormones and surgical treatments to block puberty and to fashion, as closely as possible, secondary sex characteristics that appear to match patients' "gender identity" or "gender preference."

Changing the secondary sex characteristics of people like Jules takes the PSM's rationale one step further, treating the patients' sexual organs and underlying sexual physiology as either a good to be preserved or a harm to be remedied, strictly on the basis of the patient's self-perception. In the PSM framework, in the case of Jules, who does not want male secondary sex characteristics, those characteristics are harms to him, which the physician has an obligation to remedy insofar as possible. Might the case of Jules present an opportunity to see the PSM's inadequacies? If our language and our framework of analysis lead us to think that we should block a thirteen-year-old boy's sexual maturation—often rendering the boy permanently sterile in the process—perhaps we need a new language and a new framework.

The Way of Medicine

The Way of Medicine starts with a claim that has been implicated in much of our discussion thus far. Put simply, humans, like all other animals, are organisms. Indeed, this fact makes it possible for us to recognize that bodily health is a real human good rather than an ethereal aspiration.

A corollary claim immediately follows: our existence as human animals is sexed. We are male or female organisms by virtue of having a root capacity for reproductive function, even if that capacity is immature or damaged. As with countless other species, the human reproductive function is performed jointly by two organisms of opposite sexes; no individual human being suffices for the performance of reproduction. The two sexes reflect root capacities for the general structural and behavioral patterns involved in human reproduction. In male humans, this capacity comprises the structures necessary for the production of male gametes and the performance of the male sex act, insemination. In females, the capacity comprises the structures necessary for the production of oocytes and the performance of the female sex act, reception of semen in a manner disposed to conception.

Some individuals, due to disorders of sex development, present genuine sex ambiguity. For example, females with congenital adrenal hyperplasia can be born with male-appearing external genitalia. To give another example, disorders with respect to the production and metabolism of testosterone can cause babies with male chromosomes (X, Y) to develop characteristically female external genitalia. Some sex and gender theorists have made much of these and other intersex cases in arguing that the simple binary of male and female fails to do justice to the diversity of possible sexes. And of course, opening up the number of "possible sexes" does a certain amount of work in opening up the possibility of changing one's secondary sex characteristics, which is precisely Jules's desire.[9]

Yet those who deny the sexual binary on the grounds of intersex cases ignore the distinction between paradigm cases and cases that decline from the paradigm. This distinction, recognized since Aristotle, applies to many kinds, including many kinds within the natural order.[10] Organisms, for example, come in ones: that is part of what it is to be an organism in the paradigm case. But the Hensel conjoined twins, possessing two arms and two legs but also two heads between them, are neither precisely one nor two.[11] This distinction between paradigm cases and cases that decline from the paradigm is necessary to make sense of what physicians do when they recognize congenital abnormalities, including ambiguous genitalia. Indeed, the distinction is necessary to make sense of the concept of "intersex"—that is, not clearly conforming to either the male or the female paradigm. In the same way that conjoined twins do not refute the claim that organisms are one, neither do instances of sex ambiguity refute the claim that human organisms are either male or female.

The Way of Medicine, in its orientation to patients' health, resists inducements to interfere with, interrupt, or otherwise revise the healthy development, maturation, and function of male and female sexual organs and capacities. Note that the Way of Medicine's resistance to such interventions does not depend on conclusions about normative gender expression, much less about normative sexual practices. Rather, its resistance follows directly from its orientation to health as an objective bodily good for and in human animals, male and female. Medicine operates within the boundaries required by pursuit of this good.

That being said, those who seek to change a person's sex not only contradict medicine's orientation to health but also always and necessarily fail in what they attempt. Indeed, here the logic of the PSM leads to absurd contradictions in which some justify changing secondary sex characteristics by claiming that one's phenotypic (or genetic) properties can be at odds with one's *real* sex—a feature of some disembodied reality to which only the individual has access—while others justify such interventions by claiming that there is no such thing as one's real sex.

From these mutually incompatible claims, further contradictions follow. To affirm who Jules is, we are told, physicians must reject Jules's current form and refashion his body to look very different from the body of Jules as he is. Because gender is socially constructed—not dependent on biology and anatomy—we are to change that biology and anatomy on which gender does not depend. In order to get beyond the constraints of the sexual binary, we are to reify it by seeking to produce secondary sex characteristics determined by that binary. The contradictions in such reasoning would be comical if they did not result in such tragic consequences for people like Jules.

Moreover, changes to secondary sex characteristics fall far short of bringing about a change in sex. The latter would make a male organism capable of engaging in the female sex act, or vice versa. Sex change ("gender transition") interventions do nothing of the sort. Rather, they culminate in surgeries to remove sexual organs—for example, a penis or a vagina—and to refashion simulacra of the organs that members of the opposite sex characteristically possess. But one can neither make a vagina by creating an orifice nor make a penis by creating something that becomes enlarged on stimulation. One could genuinely make a penis or a vagina only by re-creating the entire biological economy of the human being, whose development as a male or female began at conception.

Within that primordially sexed biological economy, the functions of the penis and the vagina are discernible in relation to the sexual act to which they contribute, which culminates when sperm are deposited in the vagina, where these sperm are capable of processing toward and penetrating the oocyte. Moreover, the penis and the vagina are linked intrinsically not only forward to these functions that they might eventually perform but also backward to processes, such as the production of gametes (all oocytes are produced in utero), which began many years before sexual intercourse is even possible. The biological development of male and female human organisms involves the working out through time of capacities that were present at the beginning.

Physicians can transplant a penis to a male or fashion a vagina in a female so that the organ becomes truly part of the person's biological life.[12] The situation is similar to that of a heart transplant. The organ is integrated into an organism whose biological matrix is fundamentally oriented toward that organ's presence and for whom the absence of the organ represents a significant diminishment of health. Redressing such diminishments is entirely within the scope of medicine's mandate, even if the redress does not fully restore the diminished function. For example, if a transplanted penis allows normal urination but does not result in full erectile function, it still restores a dimension of health. No surgery, however, can integrate a male sex organ into the biological life of a being whose root capacities are female (and vice versa).[13]

Unfortunately, the PSM seems increasingly committed to ignoring the antinomies and contradictions posed by granting patients the gender transition or gender affirmation interventions they seek. In doing so, the PSM makes patients' wishes and choices determinative of both sex and the purpose of medicine. Some physicians today use exogenous hormones and surgical interventions to bring about changes in patients like Jules. These changes, were they brought about in the absence of the patient's asking that they be done (or, in pediatric patients like Jules, the patient's parent asking that they be done), would be considered profound mutilations of a healthy body. So the contradictions in the PSM lead to tragic consequences, as these interventions irreversibly damage the health of the patient.[14] Yet, because these interventions are *patient-chosen*, the PSM and its surrounding social and legal culture not only permit physicians to conduct these interventions but also increasingly charge physicians who refuse to participate in them with abandoning their professional obligations to "put the patient first."[15]

The Way of Medicine cannot but dissent from these increasingly common judgments. Because the Way takes its bearings from the health of the patient as a member of the human species, the Way of Medicine sees that every surgical attempt to change an individual's sex damages or destroys some secondary sex characteristic that otherwise displays health and is necessary for reproductive function, itself a constitutive dimension of human health. This judgment of the Way of Medicine is only strengthened by the requirements of practical reason, which add a corollary concern: since sexual capacities make possible the one-flesh union of marriage, interventions that damage or destroy those capacities also prevent the realization of the basic good of marriage.

Thus, the Way of Medicine cannot countenance doing to Jules what he asks, not because of bigotry or phobia but because, in solidarity with patients like Jules, medical practitioners should act only in ways that are congruent with the patient's health and only in ways that are open to other basic goods, including marriage and child-bearing.

When a young woman with anorexia sees herself as overweight, she manifests a disorder of perception. The good physician shows no disrespect to the patient when she refuses to facilitate further weight loss through surgery or medications. Rather, such refusals are part and parcel of the physician's commitment as a physician to care for the patient. Similarly, Jules deserves our care and attention, but his problem is not the presence of male secondary sex characteristics. Rather, he suffers a disorder of perception regarding his nature as a human being, one who is irrevocably and irreducibly male. The physical harm of bodily mutilation should not compound the harms of that illusory perception.

To our minds, the willingness of contemporary medicine and society to embrace such solutions manifests one of the fullest culminations to date of the PSM to abandon concern for objective goods, to treat medicine as if it were merely technique, and to put medical technologies in service of autonomous desire. That culmination is continuous with the PSM's approach to contraception, assisted reproduction, and many other questions surrounding sexuality and reproduction that we cannot address here. It's no surprise, then, that our treatment of these issues runs radically counter to current medical orthodoxy.

Nevertheless, the Way of Medicine's approach to these issues preserves the possibility of medicine's being a profession and of medical professionals' being more than mere functionaries. The Way of Medicine also—as we show in the next chapter, on abortion—acknowledges the moral demands that a common humanity places on all of us, physicians and nonphysicians alike.

CHAPTER SEVEN

Abortion and Unborn Human Life

Let's return to the story of Cindy Parker.

Cindy received a prescription for birth control pills and took the pills consistently until she broke up with her boyfriend. She was not sure when or if she might have sex again, and one of the nurses at the student health clinic had told her that if she had unprotected sex, she could buy emergency contraception at the pharmacy without a prescription. Three months later she did have sex again, and the following morning she purchased and took emergency contraception pills. Three weeks after that, she returned to student health, having noticed that she had missed her period. A pregnancy test confirmed that she was pregnant. With tears in her eyes but determination, she asked, "Where can I get an abortion?"

No issue in medical ethics is more consequential and politically divisive than abortion, and though the legal and ethical lines have been clearly drawn for decades, political leaders, medical ethicists, clinicians, and the public alike continue to contest those lines, pushing for or against abortion restrictions.

Our goal here is not so much to trace out all of the arguments for or against abortion as to show the differences it makes if we consider Cindy's request for an abortion within the framework of the provider of services model (PSM) versus the Way of Medicine.

111

THE PROVIDER OF SERVICES MODEL

The PSM approaches a request for abortion more or less as it does a request for contraception, assisted reproduction, or gender transition. To start, the fact that abortion is constitutionally protected and is endorsed by the American College of Obstetricians and Gynecologists (ACOG) as an essential healthcare service gives Ms. Parker's request the force of law and custom.[1] In addition, autonomy again looms large in the ubiquitous language of *choice*, while beneficence again asks us to consider all of the different outcomes that Ms. Parker might have valued, with deference to Ms. Parker to decide whether abortion was the choice that would bring about the greatest good for her. The condition of nonmaleficence was satisfied in that early abortion is safe, arguably carrying less risk to Ms. Parker's health than continuing her pregnancy to term. And, once more, justice asked us to consider whether it was fair for Ms. Parker to be forced to carry to term a pregnancy that she did not want.

The language of justice has become particularly prominent among those who advocate for legal abortion. Medical students and obstetrician-gynecology residents today often receive training in "reproductive justice," a concept that makes access to the full range of family planning options an essential part of broader social justice for women and girls. If Ms. Parker was to have the same prospects that she would otherwise have had if she were male, she could not be asked to shoulder consequences that did not fall on the man with whom she had sex. Unlike him, Ms. Parker would have her life plans radically disrupted if she did not have access to abortion.

So while the PSM might acknowledge genuine moral concerns regarding abortion, it will consistently bracket them off as a matter of personal values that intrude on the clinician's professional obligation to accommodate, at least by referral, the patient's request for abortion. As long as Ms. Parker was making an apparently free and informed choice of the healthcare service she believed was best for her, her physician had to either perform the abortion or direct Ms. Parker to someone who would.

THE WAY OF MEDICINE

The question of abortion is dramatically recast in the Way of Medicine. Right up front, the Way of Medicine has us ask: what does abortion have to do with the physician's commitment to preserve and restore Ms. Parker's health? There are cases—for example, of severe pre-eclampsia or significant heart conditions—in which the condition of continued pregnancy gravely threatens the woman's health, and we return to such cases below. But in the great majority of cases, as in Ms. Parker's, abortion is sought not for the sake of health but for the sake of not having a baby. Abortion is a means of preserving current and future possibilities for the woman that appear to be threatened by carrying the pregnancy to term. That abortion concerns choice, not health, is shown by the fact that a physician will treat two otherwise identical patients differently based simply on whether their pregnancies are wanted. With one patient, the physician will celebrate the fact that she has achieved pregnancy and even promise to use all manner of medical resources to see that her pregnancy continues to term. With the other, the physician will perform or refer the patient for an abortion.

So far, then, in the Way of Medicine, physicians have good reason to decline to participate in elective abortions, quite apart from the question of what abortions do to the fetuses. In Ms. Parker's case, the physician might decline her request simply because his commitment to her as a physician does not include bringing about a state of affairs in which she is no longer pregnant.

When the life and health of the fetus are taken into account, however, the physician's refusal becomes imperative. From the time that the Hippocratic Oath was formulated until shifts in some quarters starting in the 1960s, medical oaths and codes in the West consistently condemned elective abortion as contradicting physicians' constitutive professional commitment to never intentionally damage or destroy the health and life of patients. The Hippocratic Oath stated, "I will not give to a woman an abortive remedy."[2] The "Hippocratic Oath Insofar as a Christian May Swear It," which had much wider circulation in the early centuries of the Christian era, expanded this prohibition by stating, "I will not give treatment to women to cause abortion, treatment neither from above nor from below."[3] The World Medical Association's 1948 Declaration of Geneva included the promise "I will maintain the utmost respect for human life from the time of conception, even under threat."[4]

Notably, in 1983 the words "from the time of conception, even under threat" were revised to "from its beginning, even under threat," and in 2005 these words were removed from the Declaration of Geneva altogether. These revisions were mirrored by changes in the codes of other professional associations,[5] and they reflect the fact that abortion was legalized in many countries in the later decades of the twentieth century. They also reflect, however, growing disputes about what the fetus is and whether respect for human life really rules out abortion.

Surely a fetus is not a human being, some have objected, but instead only a clump of cells. Or, even if the fetus *is* a human being, surely we do not owe to it the same kinds of treatment we owe to the human beings reading and writing this book. Moreover, what about the hard cases, in which a woman's life is in significant jeopardy? What authority do physicians, much less the state, have to tell women they should not be free to make such personal, indeed private, choices? We look at each question on the Way of Medicine.

ANIMAL ORGANISMS

Throughout this book we have presupposed that we are all animal organisms of a certain sort: human beings. The practice of medicine is founded on this truth. The vocation of the healing profession starts with a recognition that, as animal organisms, humans are susceptible to illness, disability, decline, and death. We would not need medicine if we were only disembodied souls or minds.

For complicated historical and philosophical reasons, however, modern human beings have come to think and talk about themselves as if they were souls or minds who happen to possess, for a time, a living body. Moderns are accustomed to say, for just one example, that a person suffering dementia is "not there anymore." In part, this way of talking reflects the cultural elevation of humans' singular capacity for thinking and choosing—that mindedness that seems to distinguish humans from the other animals.

Notwithstanding its popularity, this form of dualism is misguided. Pay attention to your direct experience. Right now, as you read these words, you are engaged in a sensory act, making use of your eyes and your hands, and you are oriented in space toward the physical realities of words on a page (paper or electronic); perhaps you are listening with your ears to sound vibrations in the air as the recorded book is read to you. These acts are those of a *bodily* being, specifically the organism who is sitting, reclining, or walking (with earbuds) here and now. But you are also following an argument, a train of thought, that makes use of abstract terms such as "organism" and "abstract" and "thought." These acts are those of a *minded* being, a being capable of intellection. You are both of those beings, as evidenced by your use of the word "I": "I am seeing these words on the page, and I am understanding them." Thus, the minded being you are is the same being as your physical, bodily being. One and the same being reads and understands, sees and cognizes, moves and abstracts. *You* are that human being, that living organism.

The Beginning of the Human Being

If we accept the discussion so far as true, you came into existence whenever the living organism reading this book came into existence. You were not preceded by another living human organism, as might be possible if you were a mind (or even a brain); rather, your existence commenced with the existence of the human animal reading or listening to this book right now.

When did you begin? The answer, if you are not an identical twin or a human clone, is simple: you began at fertilization, when a human sperm penetrated an oocyte and both sperm and oocyte ceased to exist, giving rise instead to a single-celled zygote. This zygote was itself a single, whole, individual member of the species *Homo sapiens*, genetically distinct from its parents and possessed of a developmental program by which it was able to execute its own growth and development to the next stages of human existence: the embryonic stage, then the fetal stage, then the infant stage, and so on.

The best evidence for this claim comes directly from the science of embryology and the authority of those who study human development and the development of other organisms, such as mice. Consider the following representative passage from K. L. Moore, T.V.N. Persaud, and Mark G. Torchia's textbook *The Developing Human: Clinically Oriented Embryology*:

> Human development begins at fertilization when a sperm fuses with an oocyte to form a single cell, the zygote. This highly specialized, totipotent cell (capable of giving rise to any cell type) marks the beginning of each of us as a unique individual. The zygote, just visible to the unaided eye, contains chromosomes and genes that are derived from the mother and father. The zygote divides many times and becomes progressively transformed into a multicellular human being through cell division, migration, growth, and differentiation.[6]

Two primary arguments are made against the claim that a human organism comes into existence at fertilization, but neither argument can be sustained. First, some claim that because the early embryo is capable of twinning, it therefore cannot be considered *one* individual organism. What shall we make of this? Does the possibility of some one thing becoming two mean that it once was not one thing? No one who has ever snapped a stick in half could believe that. Nor, in the domain of living things, are microbiologists tempted to believe that amoebae, which reproduce precisely by splitting, were not individual organisms prior to splitting. Similarly, the phenomenon of twinning does not suggest that the zygote or embryo was not a human organism prior to twinning. Rather, it indicates that some human beings came to exist later than fertilization—namely, when their embryo divided, resulting in two embryos where once there was only one.

The second argument holds that the zygote or early embryo does not have sufficient unity, within itself, to be considered a living whole.

This line of argument sees the early embryo as merely an aggregate (a "clump") of cells. Several problems arise with this claim. What could cause this mere aggregate to become one thing? Indeed, the transition of numerous cells into a single organism several days later than fertilization must be seen as an extremely implausible, inexplicable event. Moreover, embryologists find an enormous amount of activity, much of it coordinated, among the various parts of the developing embryo, activity oriented toward ensuring the embryo's survival and growth. Nor is this coordinated activity the same in all cells. Rather, embryologists observe division of labor among the cells of even the very early embryo, and from the first cell division the roles of some cells can be distinguished from the roles of others. That is, the embryo does not appear to biologists as a mere clump or aggregate of undifferentiated cells.[7]

The two claims just made—that humans are animal organisms and that human organisms begin at fertilization—concern only the way things are. They are not yet claims about ethics, about how we ought to act in light of the way things are. Yet we have said enough to demonstrate a foundational fact: abortions destroy human lives, where "human lives" means precisely the lives of actual living human beings. If medicine is committed to the health of human beings, this fact is of the greatest significance. It leads directly to the ethical claim that medical practitioners should not perform or facilitate abortions.

FULL MORAL WORTH AND RESPECT

Our discussion should also appeal to the full resources of practical reason and its requirements. In addressing abortion, we are concerned with whether killing certain human beings—namely, the unborn—is morally permissible. Could it be that as a class the unborn are excluded from the moral protection owed to other human beings? Three brief arguments can respond to this question; all have been offered in expanded form elsewhere.[8]

First, the basic human goods, including the goods of health and life, are not to be damaged or destroyed in unborn human beings any more than in born human beings. Recall our claim about basic goods:

as intrinsically good, they give us reasons to act, and intending their damage or destruction can never be reasonable. Therefore, abortion, when it involves intentionally destroying the life of an unborn human being, is always wrong, ruled out by the same principle that governs other moral absolutes. (We address below whether abortion could be something other than intentional killing.)

Next, because the basic goods of human beings are good for all, intentionally killing the unborn is unfair. As the second general requirement of practical reason, fairness was formulated with the awareness that all human beings benefit from realization of the basic goods. Full reasonableness requires, then, that we not consider the goods to be less important, or less good, in some persons than they are in others (including ourselves). Nor should we, in our pursuit of particular instances of these goods, prioritize some and neglect others on the basis of arbitrary or contingent motivations. Both of these patterns violate the Golden Rule, doing to others what we would not have them do to us.

The proponent of elective abortion who acknowledges the humanity of the unborn—who is not so self-deceived as to think of unborn human beings as mere clumps of cells—is proposing to treat the good of life and health as of lesser importance in some human beings, the unborn, than in others, and to do so on the grounds that the life of the unborn is inconvenient, unwanted, small, or an obstacle to a woman's authentic development. None of the grounds for sacrificing the lives of the unborn to privilege the lives of the born seem to us any more cogent than the grounds for privileging white lives over black, male over female, or native-born over immigrant. Fairness thus forbids us to exclude the unborn from the class of human beings who have the right not to be killed.

Finally, the right not to be killed intentionally is reasonably considered a basic or absolute right. We can distinguish between rights and protections we possess that are based on our particular contingent and sometimes changing status, condition, or circumstances, and rights we think of as absolute. The former include rights to vote, to have one's work graded on time, to be given a share in the benefits paid into in a pension system, and so on. The latter include rights not to be enslaved, raped, tortured, or killed.

The second set of rights are thought to be held always and equally by all who hold them, whomever that class includes. These rights should thus be predicated on some truth that is likewise not passing and is true equally of all who hold such rights and protections. That truth is their common humanity; being human is the characteristic that all beings who have such rights possess always and possess equally with all others who have those same rights. If that is true, the rights not to be enslaved, raped, tortured, or killed should be respected equally and always, with regard to every human being, including all unborn human beings, who are no less human than they will be once they are gestated and born.

These three arguments lead to the conclusion that what is true for medical professionals is true for all: no one should ever intentionally damage or destroy the life and health of an unborn human being. Abortion, understood as the intentional killing of an unborn human being, is always and everywhere morally impermissible.

ABORTION AND PRIVACY

These arguments also make clear that abortion is not merely a private matter. The last recourse of those who would defend abortion is to claim that arguments against it are a matter of personal, often religious, beliefs, not public or professional concern. This claim is almost never argued, but it has a kind of axiomatic quality in contemporary culture, characterized as that culture is by its emphasis on what philosopher Charles Taylor calls "the ethics of authenticity"—the notion that what is most important in life is for each person to become the self that that person authentically chooses to become, based on each individual's own lights and without the censure or imposition of external standards. This culture gives rise to the PSM.

The key premises that we have drawn upon to assess the practice of abortion, however—that human beings begin at fertilization and that all human beings have the right to not be killed at will—are neither esoteric nor a matter of religious revelation. Rather, these are claims of human reason that are accessible to all. The first is a claim of science, the second a claim of the moral law known by practical reason (natural law, the Tao). That moral law makes it possible for the public to recognize and defend human rights and to evaluate particular practices, as well as explicit policies and laws, as to whether they are just or unjust.[9]

Abortion is a public matter in a further crucial sense. When medical practitioners exclude from the scope of their concern the lives and health of some human beings, that damages the practitioners' publicly expressed commitment to patients' health. Similarly, when a polity excludes from the scope of its legal concern the lives of some human beings within its legal boundaries, that damages any publicly expressed commitment to justice and equality. These commitments are the foundations of the medical and political communities, respectively; to damage them is to damage public trust in these communities. The widespread permission, acceptance, and practice of abortion are thus public wrongs in the sense that they erode the fabric of a public, whether that public is the profession of medicine or a political state pursuing justice.

ABORTION AND INTENTION

We argued in the previous section that abortion, insofar as it involves intentional killing, is morally wrong. But must abortion always involve *intentional* killing? In chapter 5 we explained that it can be permissible to allow a bad effect if that effect is not intended, provided that proportionate reason exists for allowing it. This claim is essential for thinking about several issues surrounding abortion.

In what follows, we briefly address a famous attempt by Judith Jarvis Thomson to justify abortion by arguing that it need not involve intentional killing. We argue that in most cases abortion does involve intentional killing and that abortion for the sorts of reasons Thomson envisaged would be wrongful even if the death of the unborn were not intended.

We then turn to discuss vital conflict cases, those in which one or both of the lives of the mother and child are at mortal risk and in which one or both will surely die unless a medical intervention is performed that results in the loss of the unborn human being's life.[10] We look first at some cases in which natural law theorists exhibit wide agreement, then consider cases in which the judgment that the child's death is a side effect remains controverted.

THOMSON'S VIOLINIST

Philosopher Judith Jarvis Thomson has advanced perhaps the most famous argument in defense of abortion.[11] Thomson begins by noting that much of the debate surrounding abortion concerns whether the unborn human being is a *person*. Those who oppose abortion, she writes, typically "spend most of their time establishing that the fetus is a person, and hardly any time explaining the step from there to the impermissibility of abortion."[12] Meanwhile, "those who defend abortion rely on the premise that the fetus is not a person, but only a bit of tissue that will become a person at birth."[13] In contrast, for the purposes of her argument, Thomson grants that the fetus is a person, then asks whether abortion is indeed impermissible on that assumption. This is one of the great innovations of her article, and one reason it has gained such acclaim.

At this point, readers might note that we spent time not on the question of personhood but rather on the question of whether the fetus is a human being (a question elided in Thomson's contrast of "person" with "bit of tissue"). That the fetus is a human being we take to be a matter of settled science, but one that also can be defended philosophically. Pro-choice thinkers such as Peter Singer agree with us on this point, conceding that it is obscurantist to deny that the fetus is a human being (What else would it be?). Unlike Singer, however, we hold that it is wrong to intend the death of any human being, whereas Singer and many others hold that those human beings who do not possess certain qualities — the qualities of personhood — may be killed justifiably.

Note, then, that with respect to bioethics, and particularly the question of abortion, the language of personhood is typically invoked in order to distinguish which, among all human beings, are those who do not deserve (because they are not persons) the respect we generally owe to other human beings, including the respect of not killing them.

Our argument, then, unlike those Thomson was aware of, does not start with the idea of "person" but, in a sense, ends with it, for it follows from our conclusion that embryos and fetuses are persons, meaning beings whose lives should not be intentionally damaged or destroyed.

Thomson presents an argument for abortion that concedes this claim—that fetuses, as human beings, should not be killed *intentionally*. To do so, she presents the reader with the following scenario: You wake up to find you have been abducted by the Society of Music Lovers and medically attached to a famous violinist who is unconscious and ill. He needs the use of your kidneys for nine months to survive his disease; if you detach yourself from him, he will certainly die.

Thomson believes that the average reader will intuit that it would still be permissible to detach yourself, and in the situation as described, we agree. Thomson's scenario is one in which the rule of double effect applies. Must you, by detaching yourself, intend the death of the violinist? It seems not. Rather, you might reasonably intend to avoid the burdens of attachment. Is detaching yourself unfair? Not necessarily. In Thomson's scenario, the violinist has no real moral claim on you—you were abducted, after all—and so it does not seem unfair for you to detach yourself, thus avoiding a nine-month involuntary confinement forced on you by someone with no connection to you.

But the great majority of elective abortions do not resemble this situation at all. Like Ms. Parker, most women who seek abortions do so because they do not want, or do not feel ready, to be mothers. However understandable these desires are, in such cases the woman's intention clearly includes the death, not merely the "disconnection," of the fetus, as the fetus must die in order to prevent it from developing into a baby to whom the woman is the mother. Indeed, while Thomson believes that her argument supports only disconnection from (or, more realistically, expulsion of) the fetus, others have argued that the constitutional right to abortion in the United States entails a right to the death of the fetus lest the right to abortion be whittled away by improvements in technology that make it possible to sustain fetuses outside the womb at earlier and earlier stages of pregnancy or the right be forfeited in cases of botched abortions that produce live births.[14]

Suppose, however, that some abortions are not like this. Imagine a woman who would, if it were possible, readily permit her fetus to be removed to an external form of life support and seeks detachment merely to avoid the burdens of providing the fetus further "womb room" or sustenance. In such a case, however uncommon, detaching the fetus would not involve intentional killing, and the death of the unborn child would be a side effect. Could such an abortion be morally permissible?

Not, we suggest, in the kinds of cases Thomson has in mind. Note first the differences in the kind of relationship the reader has to the violinist compared with the relationship Ms. Parker has to the fetus inside her. In the former it may make sense to talk only of "the woman" and "the violinist," but in the latter it also makes sense to talk of "the mother" and "her child." The mother-child relationship is quite unlike the relationship between the reader and the violinist in Thomson's example, even when the mother did not desire the relationship and even, as in the tragic cases of sexual violence, when the relationship has been forced on her through another person's criminal actions. We are animal organisms, and mother and child share a real biological relationship; because those biological beings are also persons, the relationship is also personal, even if it is not desired.

We recognize that this claim will strike some as extreme, even offensive, and we readily concede that a woman who seeks an abortion after suffering sexual violence is less blameworthy than one who seeks an abortion after sexual intercourse in which she freely engaged. We also concede that when abortion is chosen to end a pregnancy that follows consensual sex, the man often bears as much responsibility for the abortion as the woman—and, in some cases, more.

The point here is not to assign blame but to clarify that, contrary to what Thomson's hypothetical would suggest, biological relationships can create obligations, even if those obligations have not been accepted voluntarily. If a young baby turns up on a man's doorstep and he realizes the baby is his biological daughter—perhaps the man had had a one-night stand and the mother has abandoned the baby—biological paternity and the child's vulnerability create a real obligation to provide assistance to the baby, one extending well beyond nine months. If the man knows that his biological daughter will surely die without the food and shelter he is able to provide, it seems to us profoundly unjust for him to refuse. The same would hold true if an elderly man showed up on the doorstep of a young woman and identified himself as her father, perhaps separated from her years before by war or another circumstance for which he was not responsible. Children never choose their biological parents, and yet it seems that children nevertheless have obligations to their parents that they do not have to others. Biological relations matter morally, even though they are not chosen. Indeed, if Thomson's violinist scenario were changed only a little—if, say, the reader learns that the violinist is the woman's long-lost child or long-lost sibling, we doubt that the reader's intuitions would be so solidly in favor of her detaching from him; indeed, they might become solidly in favor of the opposite.

In a moment, we will consider cases that differ further from Thomson's example because in them the mother's life is in danger. But we conclude here that, apart from such cases, it is typically *unjust* because unfair to refuse life-sustaining aid to one who is closely related to us, particularly when we can provide such aid and others cannot; and this unfairness is particularly at odds with a mother's unchosen vocational responsibilities. If we would help our child in the doorstep scenario or in the violinist scenario but not in the abortion scenario, it seems that our refusal to help in the abortion case is unfair—motivated by an unreasonable prejudice against the unborn. Thomson's article, then, does not in fact grant the personhood of the fetus, for it fails to treat the unborn with the respect we accord to all those whose deaths we would neither intend nor accept as a side effect without proportionate reason.

DOUBLE EFFECT AND LIFE-SAVING ABORTION

Having gone so far to critique the vast majority of abortions, we here argue that in rare cases in which a mother's life and health are gravely threatened, medical practitioners sometimes can reasonably intervene to preserve the mother's life even when their intervention will inevitably cause the death of the unborn child as a side effect. Such interventions, as we explain, neither contradict a physician's commitment to the patient's health nor are they ruled out by practical reason.

One paradigmatic such case concerns a pregnant woman with a cancerous uterus, whose cancer must be addressed before delivery or the woman will die and the child also will die. Is it permissible to perform a hysterectomy on the woman, removing the cancerous uterus and with it the unborn, pre-viable child, even though this inevitably will result in the child's death? The rule of double effect indicates that the answer is yes: the end of the surgery is preserving the mother's life; the means is the removal of her diseased uterus. The bad effect, which it would be immoral to intend, is the death of the unborn human being. Is there a proportionately good reason to accept that effect? In this case, yes, clearly: both mother and child will die if the operation is not performed. Thus no one is being privileged, much less arbitrarily privileged, over another. The mother's life is not judged more important than the child's; rather, her life is the only life that can be saved. In this case, the Way of Medicine would approve of the hysterectomy.

What if the life of the mother could be preserved, or that of the child, but not both? Some argue that the mother's life should be preserved over the child's because the mother is the physician's primary patient. To us this conclusion does not seem obvious. A physician charged with caring for a pregnant woman has, whether he recognizes it or not, two patients—two vulnerable persons under his care whose health is at stake. Those persons stand in somewhat different relationships to the physician, for only one can communicate her wishes and decisions, agree to be the physician's patient, and so on. But, as in the case of a traffic accident that a doctor happens upon, we think that the proximity of the vulnerable child and the exigency of the child's health-related needs—not to mention the child's relatedness to the physician's obvious patient—both contribute, in conjunction with the physician's vocation, to the physician's having obligations directly to the child in addition to the child's mother.

That being said, the woman, as the child's mother, has substantial authority to make decisions both for herself and for her child. She is the one in the position to evaluate the options in light of her own vocation. Although in principle either decision could be fair, her vocational commitments and obligations give her reasons in light of which she can determine which choice to make in this awful situation.[15] In our view, therefore, the decision as to whether the physician should strive to preserve her life or the life of her child is the mother's to make.

A salpingectomy for an ectopic pregnancy is another paradigmatic scenario in which the Way of Medicine permits a lethal intervention. In such a case, the embryo has implanted in the woman's fallopian tube. Continued pregnancy will inevitably lead to the death of the embryo, and it also can threaten the life of the mother if the fallopian tube ruptures. In a salpingectomy, the surgeon removes the portion of the fallopian tube that contains the embryo. Again, the physician's end is to preserve the mother's life and health; the means is removing the compromised segment of the fallopian tube. Negative effects of this intervention include not only the embryo's death but also the risk of future infertility in the woman. This case seems to straightforwardly satisfy the rule of double effect, along the same lines as the case of the woman with a gravid but cancerous uterus.

Before turning to more contentious cases, let's consider the definition of "abortion." Earlier we argued that it is always impermissible to intentionally kill an unborn human being. We then, in response to Judith Jarvis Thomson's line of reasoning, argued that in the great majority of cases it is also impermissible, because unfair, to accept the death of the unborn child as a side effect of an intervention to end the state of pregnancy. However, the two cases we have just described—those of the pregnant woman with cancer in her uterus and the woman with an ectopic pregnancy—both indicate that in some cases a physician can intervene to preserve the mother's life and health even when doing so will inevitably cause the death of an unborn human being.

So we propose to define "abortion" not as any medical intervention that results in the death of an unborn human being but rather as *any act that either intentionally or unjustly ends the life of an unborn human being.* All abortion so defined is morally impermissible, and likewise, no act is an abortion that accepts the death of an unborn human being as the justifiable side effect of an attempt to preserve the mother's life.

CONTROVERSIAL CONFLICT CASES

In this section we briefly discuss three cases that continue to be controversial among proponents of the Way of Medicine. Although we cannot settle these cases definitively, we show how the controversy surrounding them illustrates the two different approaches to intention that we described in chapter 5. In each case, the debate concerns whether the death of the unborn human being is intended or is a side effect.

The Phoenix Case

In 2009 a dispute arose concerning whether an attempt to save a mother's life was an abortion or a justified application of the rule of double effect. The case occurred in Phoenix, Arizona, and the hospital in question described it thus:

> A woman in her 20s with a history of moderate but well-controlled pulmonary hypertension found out she was pregnant. There was concern for her health, because pregnancy with pulmonary hypertension carries a serious risk of mortality. Because of the severity of her disease, the woman's risk of mortality was close to 50 percent. In November 2009, the woman was admitted to St. Joseph's Hospital and Medical Center with worsening symptoms. Tests revealed that she now had life-threatening pulmonary hypertension. The chart notes that she had been informed that her risk of mortality was close to 100% if she continued the pregnancy. The medical team contacted the Ethics Consult team for review. The consultation team talked to several physicians and nurses as well as reviewed the patient's record. The patient and her family, her doctors, and the Ethics Consult team agreed that the pregnancy could be terminated and that it was appropriate since the goal was not to end the pregnancy but to save the mother's life.[16]

How does one analyze this case with respect to the intention of the mother and her doctors? In chapter 5 we distinguished between two accounts of intention. For one, what matters primarily is what is proposed and undertaken from the standpoint of the agent who is acting. For the other, external factors such as closeness bear on what an agent intends. In the first account, from the standpoint of the mother and the physicians, the fetus's death is not the means by which the strain on her heart may be relieved; the means, rather, is removal of the connection between her child and her body. The placental connection to the fetus is putting inordinate strain on her heart, thus gravely threatening her health and life, and removing that connection is itself the action necessary to preserve her life. So, in this first account, the death of the fetus is not intended. We still need to consider whether there was proportionate reason to allow the death of the fetus as a side effect and, in particular, whether allowing that death was fair given that the child was going to die no matter what was done. We return to this question shortly.

But first, consider the following analysis advanced by Fr. Nicanor Austriaco, which is emblematic of the alternative account of intention:

> When the doctors chose to remove the child's placenta to save his mother's life, they necessarily also chose to kill him, because they were choosing to remove a vital organ of an innocent human being in a manner that would end his life. They chose to kill him in the same way that a Mayan priest who chooses to remove a beating heart from a sacrificial victim to placate the gods also chooses to kill him. Evil was done (the killing of the child) for the sake of obtaining a good (the restoration of the health of the mother).[17]

On Austriaco's understanding of intention, to choose to "remove a vital organ" (the placenta) is choosing to kill, regardless of how things are understood from the agent's perspective. Accordingly, the question is settled immediately: intentional killing is always wrong, so the doctors' actions in the Phoenix case were unethical.

We disagree with Fr. Austriaco's analysis. The death of the fetus accomplished nothing for the mother or the physicians. Rather it was entirely the detachment of the placenta that was sought, and then the subsequent removal of the placental and fetal remains. We do not think it accurate to say that "they necessarily also chose to kill [the fetus]." Rather, they chose to detach the placenta, foreseeing and accepting that the fetus would be killed as a side effect.

There remains the question of whether this decision was fair, and here we think the answer is clear. If the death was not intended, the decision to end the pregnancy was certainly fair, as otherwise both lives would have been lost. The intervention did not privilege one life over another but merely preserved one life instead of sacrificing both. We think it evident that the intervention honored the Golden Rule—that a reasonable person, faced with a scenario in which both the child and his mother would die soon if nothing were done, but in which his mother's life might be preserved by a procedure that would result in his death, would affirm the intervention to preserve his mother's life. This is not unlike an awful scenario in which one rock climber who has fallen is hanging tethered to another, and both will die unless the tether is cut. If the agent-centered account of intention is correct, and if neither the mother nor her doctors intended her baby's death, the placentectomy was not an abortion and was instead a properly health-motivated intervention, albeit one with a tragic consequence.

Ectopic Complications

Among proponents of the Way of Medicine, similar disagreements have persisted about how to address ectopic pregnancies. As we noted, salpingectomy is universally supported, but questions have been raised about two alternate interventions, salpingotomy and administration of the drug methotrexate.

In a salpingotomy, a longitudinal incision is made in the fallopian tube, and the embryo is flushed out using a suction-irrigator. Obstetricians have generally preferred salpingotomy over salpingectomy because it has been thought that salpingotomy would better preserve the woman's fertility, though that intuition has not been born out in clinical studies.[18] Meanwhile, the direct physical connection between the intervention and the embryo's death has convinced some that the latter must be intended as part of the former. Certainly, the connection to the embryo's death is not as indirect as it is in a salpingectomy.

Directness or indirectness, however, has no necessary bearing on whether an effect is intended or not. Indeed, in the first philosophical treatment of double effect, Thomas Aquinas argued that lethal force could sometimes be used in self-defense. To us, the use of a sword to fend off an attacker has a similarly direct connection to the resulting injury or death the attacker suffers.

Moreover, it seems clear that the embryo's death is generally not part of the mother's or the physicians' proposals. Rather, their proposals are to preserve the mother's health and life by removing the embryo from a place where it threatens grave danger to the mother. While the embryo's death is indeed an inevitable consequence, it is not needed as a means; presumably, if the physicians could move the embryo to the uterus without harm, they would. If that is true, as long as there is a proportionate reason to accept the death of the embryo, as there seems clearly to be on the same grounds we discussed with respect to salpingectomy, a salpingotomy is permissible.

Finally, there is the question of treating an ectopic pregnancy with the drug methotrexate. This drug inhibits cell division in the trophoblast, which is the precursor to the placenta. In an ectopic pregnancy, the trophoblast cells burrow into the cells of the fallopian tube, as they would into the endometrial lining of the uterus in a healthy pregnancy. By preventing cell division in the trophoblast, methotrexate prevents the embryo from remaining attached to the fallopian tube; without maintaining this attachment, the embryo dies.

Again one can see why proponents of a less agent-centered account of intention conclude that the use of methotrexate involves intentional killing: the drug inhibits cell division not only in the trophoblast but also in the embryo as a whole. Moreover, the trophoblast is part of the embryo, so it seems again that the intervention directly attacks the embryo even if the agent aims to affect only the trophoblast.

On the other hand, from the agent's perspective, it seems that the aim is to preserve the mother's health and the means is detachment, which is achieved by inhibiting the trophoblast cells specifically. The overall lethal effect is not part of the proposal and thus not intended.

We may seem to be splitting hairs, but a question looms here that is hard to settle: when an intended effect is part of a larger whole that is caused in order to bring about the effect, is that whole itself intended? Elizabeth Anscombe raised this question in relation to a case in which the Allies bombed Dutch dikes to flood the Zeelands and thereby kill German soldiers. Many Zeelanders were also killed, and the question Anscombe raised is this: were they killed as side effects of an effort that targeted only the Germans, or were the Germans killed as part of an effort to kill *everyone* by means of the flooding? With respect to the use of methotrexate for ectopic pregnancy, is the loss of cell division throughout the embryo a side effect of an effort to block such division only in the trophoblast, or does the agent intend to inhibit the cell division of the embryo as a whole in order to inhibit cell division in the trophoblast? If the latter, the agent seems to make the embryo's death the means to the embryo's detachment rather than accepting it as a side effect of that detachment. Then the use of methotrexate appears to be an instance of a chemical rather than a surgical abortion.[19]

Conclusion

As we noted at the outset of this chapter, we cannot do justice here to all of the arguments for and against abortion. Instead, we have aimed to show, first, that abortion not only falls outside the proper scope of the medical profession but that it contradicts that profession's commitment to never intentionally damage or destroy the life and health of any human being. In addition, we gave reasons for thinking that a stronger conclusion is true: that no one should ever intend the death of an unborn human being, nor should they accept such a death as the foreseen side effect of unjustly refusing to give aid to an unborn human being. Finally, we showed that the rule of double effect is essential to practical reasoning about hard cases: cases in which one or both of the lives of a mother and her child will be lost in the absence of an intervention that itself has lethal effects.

This concludes our treatment of medical ethics at the beginning of life. We turn now to the practice of medicine and medical ethics at life's end.

CHAPTER EIGHT

Medicine at the End of Life

Now let's return to the story of Abe Anderson and look further into that of Nora Garcia.

Abe has been found to have advanced cancer.

Nora has suffered a devastating stroke.

In this chapter we will examine the ethical questions that arise in caring for patients with advanced illness or those who are at the end of life. Most clinical ethics consultations are called to address such questions, which is natural enough, given the two kinds of limits we face. First, we face the limits imposed by human mortality. Aging happens; health declines irrevocably. The health that can be restored is less than it once was. Losses abound; death looms. These limits raise this question: how does one appropriately pursue health when health is irreversibly diminishing?

Second, we face the related limits of medicine. Medicine cannot reverse aging. It cannot overcome the fact that all of us will die, relatively soon. So medicine's efforts become more strenuous and burdensome in exchange for less substantial gains. More is wagered, but less is accomplished. Leon Kass memorably wrote, "Health is a mortal good, and . . . we are fragile beings that must snap sooner or later, medicine or no medicine. To keep the strings in tune, not to stretch them out of shape attempting to make them last forever, is the doctor's primary and proper goal."[1]

Since the advent of the mechanical ventilator, however, physicians, patients, and family members have come to experience the default pathway for dying in American healthcare precisely as a process of being stretched out of shape by life-sustaining technology in a vain attempt to postpone death as long as possible. Unfortunately, out of otherwise reasonable desires that death and the suffering that accompanies it not be unreasonably prolonged, some have moved to embrace death itself as one of the ends of medicine, as if destroying the instrument were the best means of tuning the strings.

What would it look like merely to keep the strings in tune or at least in such tune as is available? And why is destroying the life of a patient not a solution to the problem of the patient's strings being stretched out of shape? In this chapter we address the first of these questions, and in chapter 9 the second.

SEEKING THE HEALTH THAT IS POSSIBLE

Abe Anderson and his wife undergo in vitro fertilization, and two years later they are the proud parents of twin girls. One day Abe's wife notices that his eyes look yellow. Abe returns to his doctor. Radiographic imaging reveals a tumor in his pancreas, with multiple lesions in his liver. A procedure is done to place a stent in Abe's bile duct, and biopsies confirm what everyone fears: he has metastatic pancreatic cancer.

What should the doctor suggest in the face of Abe's diagnosis? How should Abe discern a reasonable way forward? We have proposed that the end of medicine is health; what could it mean to pursue the health of a patient whose disease is incurable? What health-related options are available to someone in Abe's tragic but not uncommon situation?

For simplicity's sake, suppose that Abe's physician believes she can present Abe with two options. We want to ask, first, are these options genuinely permissible for a doctor vocationally committed to health, and second, how should Abe deliberate about these options practically?

Option 1 is to undergo a regimen of chemotherapy. Clinical studies indicate that patients like Abe who receive this regimen live only a month longer, on average, and many die sooner than they otherwise would have, but about one in five patients survive at least a year. Major side effects of this regimen include nausea, vomiting, fatigue, anemia, and immune suppression.

Option 2 is to focus on palliation—treating Abe's pain and other symptoms as they arise and working to sustain his remaining health and function using interventions that are not particularly burdensome, but forgoing further cancer-directed treatment. Often a palliative approach is structured under hospice care. Clinical studies indicate that patients like Abe who choose Option 2 will live about as long, on average, as those who receive chemotherapy. However, almost all such patients die within a year.

Consider how this decision would be framed under the provider of services model (PSM). First, physicians and patients would consider the universe of options that are technically possible, permitted by current law and professional standards, and available in the patient's context. The conventional approach would not hold these options up against a specific end or norm, such as the patient's health. The patient and the clinician would thus not be accountable to an objective standard, although they would still have resources for discernment. They could apply the four principles of bioethics—autonomy, beneficence, nonmaleficence, and justice. Alternatively, they could try to put the known benefits and harms of the two approaches onto some kind of scale to determine which course of action would bring about the greatest good for the greatest number, or at least bring about the greatest good for Abe.

Under the PSM, the resolution of the matter ultimately defaults to the patient's wishes. No one but the patient, after all, is in a position to weigh all of these considerations against the subjective norm of the patient's well-being—the state of affairs that the patient judges to be most desirable, that most aligns with the way the patient authentically chooses to live. In this light, Abe might reasonably choose Option 1 because it would maximize the likelihood of his being alive in a year, a state of affairs he highly values, and because it would align with his identity as a "fighter" — someone who is not going to roll over and surrender to cancer. His physician might go along because she believes that treating the cancer aligns with the principle of beneficence and that doing what Abe requests respects his autonomy.

Abe might choose Option 2 because he believes it would maximize the likelihood that he could avoid pain and other symptoms or at least they could be adequately treated. Being without pain is another state of affairs he highly values, ensuring that he would have a decent quality of life and could continue for as long as possible to do the things that make him who he is. His physician might support this approach because it seems to align with the principle of nonmaleficence and, again, to honor Abe's autonomy. Either way, the goal is for Abe to make a choice that is free, informed, and authentic to his self-perception. A choice that meets these criteria would be made ethically, irrespective of what is chosen.

To summarize, under the PSM the physician offers the range of legally permitted and medically available options, and the patient autonomously chooses the options that comport with his or her own subjective sense of *well-being*.

Interestingly, the Way of Medicine offers guidance that seems to overlap considerably with the PSM approach, although crucial differences distinguish the two. In the first place, options and choices that seem unmotivated by anything other than conventional expectations and subjective preferences under the PSM are given objective guidance in the Way of Medicine. Second, the objective norms that practitioners of the Way of Medicine apply here, where the two approaches overlap, result in very different guidance further down the line when patients are reaching for last-resort options.

THE PHYSICIAN'S OPTIONS

The Way of Medicine begins with health and with the physician's orientation toward the health that still can be preserved and restored in the patient. Abe's dire situation calls for some reminders about what health is and what it is not; practitioners must not lose this orientation. Health is not the absence of disease. If it were, the good of health would no longer be available to Abe, and his physician would have nothing more to do. Nor is health a matter of black-and-white. Clearly Abe's health will be forever diminished by pancreatic cancer; speaking colloquially, we might say that Abe will never again be healthy. Yet much health remains for Abe, and until his last breath he will enjoy some measure of it, however diminished and unsatisfactory.

Further, health is complex in its dimensions. Abe's physician rightly has in mind Abe's health as a whole organism, given our definition of health as "the well-working of the whole." But the complexity of the whole means that different dimensions of health are at stake in clinical decisions, and pursuit of one dimension often has adverse consequences for another dimension. In addition, health is a basic human good but not the only or even the highest good. As such, at the outset we know that ignoring health or certain dimensions of health makes sense under some conditions. Abe's physician needs to be mindful of these conditions.

The threshold question for a physician—the one that sets out the universe of options to consider—is which, among the technically feasible courses of action, are those plausibly conducive to the patient's health? In this framework, Option 1, the regimen of chemotherapy, can reasonably be offered only insofar as it aims at and has some probability of preserving or restoring the patient's health. Does it?

With Option 1, there is no clear answer. If the chemotherapy would increase by only 1 percent Abe's probability of living for one year, the answer would more obviously be no. If it increased that probability to 50 percent, that answer might obviously be yes. But in the case as it is, Abe's physician must make use of her prudential medical judgment: does this regimen offer a sufficiently realistic possibility of benefit that pursuing it would not be pointless? If Abe's physician believes a regimen is pointless, she does her patient no real service by offering the option. The offer would waste her patient's time, money, and energy and would subject him to other negative effects.

We think Abe's physician could reasonably judge Option 1 a live option in terms of its potential health benefits, but what about its harms: anemia and immune suppression, not to mention nausea, vomiting, and fatigue? How can Abe's physician reasonably inflict these harms on Abe? How can she cause harm to Abe's health without contradicting her profession, and what would give her sufficient reason for doing so?

According to the Way of Medicine, the physician should never intentionally harm or destroy Abe's health. Certain options are simply off the table. But the rule of double effect teaches that Abe and his physician might reasonably accept injuries to health or other goods when those injuries are foreseen but unintended side effects of pursuing Abe's health. As such, Option 1 could be reasonable from the physician's standpoint insofar as the anemia, nausea, and so on were not part of her intention. Some observers would argue that we dissimulate here, that it is nonsense to say that the physician does not intend the immune suppression, nausea, and so on when she knows with certainty that such harms result from a course of chemotherapy. But a good physician might administer Option 1 with the intention of destroying cancer cells and thereby improving the patient's health, not intending to cause nausea or anemia. That the latter are not part of the physician's intention is made clear by the observation that, for example, if the patient does not experience nausea, the physician would not consider herself to have failed (although she might wonder whether the drug was administered correctly).

What about Option 2? How could it be reasonable for a physician— whose commitment is to her patient's health—to offer or participate in a palliative approach to illness that seems to be detached from the pursuit of Abe's health? How could it be reasonable to forgo treatments that might extend Abe's life or, in other cases, even cure the patient? How can one hold, as does the Way of Medicine, that palliative medicine is oriented toward rather than abandoning patients' health?

Thinking of palliation as oriented to health can certainly seem strange. Isn't palliative care pursued, after all, precisely when health can no longer be restored, as in Abe's case? This way of thinking, however, misidentifies health as the absence of disease. One cannot capture all the dimensions of Abe's health by focusing only on his cancer. Nor is health the only good that Abe has in view. So while Abe might, as we will see below, reasonably choose not to pursue aggressive treatment of his cancer—perhaps because of commitments to other basic goods—his physician can still maintain a commitment to his health in dimensions other than the fact of his cancer. Put another way, palliative medicine is indeed good medicine for a patient like Abe, as we will address in greater detail below.

Authority manifests in Abe's situation as follows: Under the PSM, authority is vested, in the guise of patient autonomy, almost exclusively in the patient. Abe has the authority to choose among the universe of options that are technically feasible, legal (and not prohibited by professional policy), and available in his context. The physician's authority is rather limited. She is authorized to refuse interventions that are technically infeasible, illegal, or unavailable, and she retains the authority to refuse interventions that are futile in relation to the patient's goals. For example, the physician might refuse a chemotherapy regimen that clinical trials do not support. By habit and residual convention, at least to this point, physicians also generally retain the authority to refuse to participate in interventions that cause major direct harm to their patients' health, particularly when the prospects of a proportionate health benefit are doubtful. If Abe begins to suffer severe immune suppression, the physician might stop his chemotherapy regimen, even if Abe wants to continue. Although this authority of refusal continues at present as a matter of convention, such refusals may not make sense within the PSM insofar as they suggest an objective standard for harms and benefits that the framework denies. Physicians' refusals appear rather to be a holdover—one of many—from the Way of Medicine that will increasingly come to seem an arbitrary imposition of the physician's judgment regarding what the patient should value.

In the Way of Medicine the physician retains the authority to decide which courses of action sufficiently conduce to the patient's health and thereby cohere with the medical profession. Perhaps Abe has read about an experimental treatment that his physician believes poses too much risk to health with too little prospect of benefit. She exercises her authority justly when she refuses to offer such treatment. Recall, however, that the Way of Medicine does not limit physicians to one course of action that maximizes health. Among the options plausibly conducive to the patient's health, the physician has good reason to recommend the one that she believes is best, all things considered, while taking into account the patient's input. Typically no one "best" option is available, however, even in terms of health outcomes, so the patient has the authority to decide among the physician's proposals. A physician can be both too accommodating, cooperating in medical practices that are not congruent with her commitment to health, and too scrupulous, mandating the course of action that the physician believes is best rather than offering patients a choice among reasonable options.

THE PATIENT'S OPTIONS

We can't forget the patient's perspective. How should Abe think of the options his physician has presented? Our answer consolidates much that we have already discussed and introduces two terms that help us to further explain the Way of Medicine.

The starting point for Abe's deliberations is that he should not intentionally damage or destroy any basic good, including the good of life and health. Any choice he makes among the options presented to him, however, will result in some damage to the basic good of health. Option 1 risks an earlier death and will cause Abe to suffer the negative side effects of chemotherapy. Option 2 will forego the opportunity to potentially prolong his life and advance his health, even if only temporarily.

In light of the information available to him, Abe must determine whether he can reasonably pursue the associated benefits and accept the associated burdens of these options. He must ask, in other words, whether the benefits he would seek are proportionate to the burdens he must accept, or, alternatively, whether the harms he would avoid are proportionate to the benefits he must forego. This familiar practical scenario requires Abe to apply the rule of double effect. If Abe chooses uprightly, the negative consequences of his choices will always be side effects.

In making clinical choices, patients like Abe face burdens that extend beyond negative effects on health, including losses of time and money, as well as losses of other opportunities. The patient also may experience emotional aversions and repugnances toward an intervention, if, for example, it leads to hair loss, fatigue, incontinence, or impotence. Abe must consider all of these factors as he weighs his options, but by what standard is he to evaluate them?

The fitting standard in our view is his vocation. Abe is a husband and a parent of two small girls. His life situation is considerably different from, say, that of Mrs. Garcia, an elderly woman whose situation we consider later in the chapter. Abe has work obligations and debts. Perhaps he is alienated from certain friends or family members. Maybe he is a religious man, or perhaps he has let his religious life drift and feels estranged from God. All these considerations must be brought to bear on his options to determine which best fit his range of vocational commitments and responsibilities.

Sometimes a patient will judge all of the treatment options compatible with his or her station in life. In that case, in a sense, not much hangs on the patient's choice. But in many cases, some treatment options are ruled out as incompatible with the patient's vocation. Abe might, for example, judge that for him the benefits of Option 1 are simply not proportionate to its burdens. If so, we could say, using language traditional to the Way of Medicine, that for him Option 1 is *extraordinary*. Those options that he judges acceptable, in contrast, we can call *ordinary*. An extraordinary treatment should not be chosen; an ordinary treatment may be and sometimes must be chosen—if, for example, it is required by his vocation.

Some proponents of the Way of Medicine might object that our view here seems like a version of the PSM, with its emphasis on patient choice, well-being, and authenticity. We disagree. Although patient vocation is a relative standard, it is not subjective. Presuming that he is clear-thinking and reasonable, Abe uniquely understands his own vocation, and he forms his judgments of what is ordinary and extraordinary in relation to that vocation. Moreover, judging in accordance with one's vocation is judging authentically and autonomously, but Abe's judging autonomously is not sufficient for moral rightness, for Abe can judge wrongly that some option is consistent with, called for by, or incompatible with his vocation.

Consider, for example, that the palliative option offers him the most quality time with his family and the clearest mind with which to face his impending death. Perhaps it will also be too financially and emotionally taxing for his young family to accompany Abe on the path of chemotherapy, especially when the benefits are so tenuous. So let us suppose that Abe, consistent with his vocation, chooses the palliative care option. Making such a choice requires some real virtues: wisdom, to recognize that it is the right choice, and courage, to face the hard truth that he will likely be dead within a short period of time. Virtue being always in short supply, Abe will face abundant temptations to choose something that (we are stipulating) offers only a false hope and only the appearance of fighting. That Abe has the authority to make such a choice does not make his choice right. Even here, despite apparent similarities, the Way of Medicine differs fundamentally from the PSM.

THE RELIEF OF SUFFERING

Before going further, let's return to a question raised by Option 2, the prospect of a palliative approach to Abe's illness. Palliative medicine treats pain and other symptoms, thereby reducing suffering. What does reducing suffering have to do with medicine—that is, with the patient's health?

As mentioned earlier, by forgoing medical interventions that are burdensome and time-consuming, a palliative approach leaves more room for a patient to pursue other worthy goods—whether work, play, worship, or simply putting one's affairs in order before dying. In this sense, a palliative approach is justified insofar as it avoids the mistake of treating health as if it were the only or the highest good. Palliative medicine goes further, of course, by treating pain and other causes of suffering.

But this key objection remains: the notion that palliative medicine aims at health seems counterintuitive, because it seems that we deploy palliative medicine when health can no longer be restored, when diseases are incurable. This intuitive way of thinking, we propose, misunderstands health as well as the practices of palliative medicine. Again, health is not merely the absence of disease. It is, as Leon Kass put it, the "well-working of the organism as a whole," manifest in the activity of the body "in accordance with its specific excellences." Kass pointed to a squirrel to illustrate health. A squirrel's health is displayed in its characteristic activities of well-working, such as burying nuts, chattering, and climbing trees. The characteristic activities of humans are more varied, of course, and so therefore are their expressions of health, but such expressions certainly include the capacity to eat and digest food without vomiting it up, to move one's bowels, to sit or lie or walk without wracking pain, and to stay awake and fall asleep at the proper times. Palliative medicine cannot return Abe to the state of health he had before his diagnosis, but if it helps him go from a state of nausea, constipation, insomnia, and wracking pain to one in which he is able to tolerate food, move his bowels, sleep six hours at night, and move around free of debilitating pain, palliative medicine will have contributed to Abe's health. These sorts of contributions to health make it possible for Abe to pursue other goods still available to him.

Here the distinction between the PSM and the Way of Medicine begins to have practical and not just theoretical consequences. Palliating disabling symptoms with an eye to preserving and restoring a measure of health differs fundamentally from palliating symptoms without respect to whether doing so will restore health. Physicians should respect this distinction, embracing the former practices of palliation and resisting the latter.

The PSM, however, treats this distinction as clinically and ethically insignificant, urging pursuit only of that state of affairs that the patient values or desires. By this standard, only coldhearted and unreasonable doctors would refuse interventions that would end a patient's suffering simply because those interventions might contradict medicine's traditional orientation to health. What good does this narrow focus on health do for a patient dying of cancer?

In the environment of the PSM, "palliative care" has come to be cast as a broader, more holistic, more comprehensive form of professionalized care than mere medicine can offer. In effect, rather than being an essential practice within medicine, palliative care becomes an alternative and rival to medicine, with more expansive goals. For example, the World Health Organization defines "palliative care" as "an approach that improves the quality of life of patients and their families facing the problems associated with life-threatening illness through the prevention and relief of suffering by means of early identification and impeccable assessment and treatment of pain and other problems, physical, psychosocial, and spiritual."[2]

This formulation gives palliative care a seemingly boundless scope of activity. What problems, after all, are excluded from the categories of physical, psychosocial, and spiritual? In this formulation, the goal is not restoring health per se, but rather relieving suffering and improving a patient's quality of life. That goal is to be achieved through assessment and treatment—concepts that resonate with the vocabulary of medicine—yet neither suffering nor quality of life is necessarily related to health.

When efforts to relieve suffering and improve quality of life become unhinged from the goals of preserving and restoring health, palliative practitioners begin to see all forms of suffering as conditions that call for treatment, including existential suffering. Furthermore, because palliative care is committed to maximizing patient control, and because only the sufferer can authoritatively assess suffering and quality of life, palliative care practitioners trade clinical judgment oriented to the patient's health for the direction given by patient preferences. Indeed, palliative professionals are often encouraged to relieve conditions on the basis of the patient's considering the condition "unacceptable" or "intolerable," setting aside the physician's judgment regarding how the condition or its treatment is health-related.[3]

Ultimately, in order to minimize suffering and maximize quality of life, and to do so according to patients' values, physicians come to consider death itself, albeit a "good death," as one of their goals. The National Hospice and Palliative Care Organization describes "hospice" as follows: "Hospice affirms the concept of palliative care as an intensive program that enhances comfort and promotes the quality of life for individuals and their families. When cure is no longer possible, hospice recognizes that a peaceful and comfortable death is an essential goal of health care."[4] In this formulation, palliative care shifts from relieving disabling symptoms so that patients can live as well as possible in the face of death to treating unwanted symptoms so that patients can die comfortably. It shifts from helping patients who are dying to helping patients to die.

No wonder that recent years have witnessed a groundswell of support for "last-resort options" in palliative care, including physicians' helping their patients to die via suicide and euthanasia. These last-resort options are the focus of chapter 9.

The Loss of Decision-Making Capacity

Nora Garcia is an eighty-year-old woman with a history of diabetes, high blood pressure, and coronary artery disease. At the encouragement of her geriatrician, Mrs. Garcia wrote a living will in which she stated that if she were in an irreversible coma, she would not want to be kept alive. She also told her physician in a conversation that he documented that she never wanted to be stuck on a breathing machine. "Just let me go," she said. One day Mrs. Garcia develops a fever, chills, cough, breathlessness, and confusion. By the time an ambulance delivers her to the local emergency room, she is found to be on the brink of respiratory failure from pneumonia.

Mrs. Garcia's case brings to light the common phenomenon of patients who are not able to make medical decisions for themselves. Young children do not have the capacity to make their own medical decisions, and even older children, for the most part, lack authority under the law to make medical decisions. Adults, however, are expected to be self-determining, and as people age many fear that they will be treated in ways they do not want—either receiving more medical interventions than they desire in the default pathway for technological medicine or receiving less medical support than they believe they deserve. In his best-selling book *Being Mortal*, physician-author Atul Gawande lamented the fact that despite handwringing all around, patients continue to suffer and die in ways that depart from what they say they would want, and contemporary medicine bears much of the blame.[5]

The problem is not that patients are receiving medical interventions that they actively refuse. Rather, the default pathway moves people inexorably toward life-sustaining technology that, when people are in better health, many would not imagine wanting. When people lose the capacity to make decisions for themselves, they often remain on that default pathway, continuing to receive interventions that they did not desire when healthy, and still would not desire.

The PSM has sought to address this problem by shoring up patients' autonomy, ensuring that medical care at the end of life accords more fully with patients' wishes. The primary mechanism for bolstering patients' autonomy, and the one that has received the most public attention and encouragement, is advance directives. *Advance directives* permit patients to specify, in writing, what kinds of medical treatment they would want if they were to suffer injuries or other health losses in the future. A living will (which Mrs. Garcia had) sets out in writing what kind of medical treatments one would want. Increasingly, physician orders for life-sustaining treatment (POLST) are used to specify these wishes and give them authority within health care. A durable power of attorney for health care (DPOAHC) specifies who is authorized to make health care decisions for the patient if the patient cannot make decisions for himself. Different advance directives carry different levels of legal authority, depending partly on where the patient lives, but all of them become active when a patient loses decisional capacity. In theory, advance directives ensure that patients' autonomy is respected when patients cannot exercise that autonomy. In practice, advance directives help to mitigate the pattern that Gawande and others have observed, in which patients who lose decisional capacity cannot get off the train that leads to unwanted and unhelpful medical interventions.

A number of criticisms have been raised regarding advance directives. The first is that they do not genuinely protect or further autonomy. Mrs. Garcia, when she wrote her living will, could not have anticipated the particular situation in which she is now, and now that she is in this situation, she does not have any autonomy. She still deserves respect, but her autonomy cannot command our respect when her illness has removed that autonomy.

The emergency room physicians face an urgent question: should they intubate Ms. Garcia to support her breathing while they give her fluids, antibiotics, and other ministrations in hopes of restoring her to the health she had before this infection? Or should they forgo the ventilator in light of her statement that she would not want to be kept alive on a breathing machine, knowing that without the ventilator she likely will not survive the next twenty-four hours?

The PSM emphasizes the subjective norm: what would she have wanted? The problem is that her physicians cannot know, because Mrs. Garcia herself could not know, what she would want in this particular situation. She certainly didn't envisage this scenario when she wrote her living will. With an unclear advance directive—and most living wills are similarly unclear—physicians typically turn to duly authorized surrogate decision-makers. While we address surrogates in a moment, let's assume at this point in the story that no such surrogates are available. In the conventional approach, in light of uncertainty about what the patient would have wanted, the physicians might do what most people want them to do in such cases—that is, what people who have the capacity to choose typically choose: they would intubate Mrs. Garcia to see if they could turn her illness around. Such decisions are sometimes justified on the grounds that they restore the patient to a state in which she can make a more considered, authentically autonomous, choice. Dying, of course, cuts off all possibilities of future autonomy.

On the Way of Medicine, Mrs. Garcia's physicians have good reason to act expeditiously to maintain the health that can be preserved using reasonable means. This aligns with the constitutive purpose of medicine—a predisposition to preserve health when possible. This disposition reasonably accepts that health is a basic good for an eighty-year-old, just as for a twenty-five-year-old; age can limit what health is possible but not the goodness of health itself.

As we have stressed, health is not the only good, and actions available to restore health have limits. Therefore, physicians need not do everything possible to keep Mrs. Garcia alive, as if there were no other goods at stake, and they need not do anything that is clearly either excessively burdensome or unlikely to preserve or restore a significant measure of health. These judgments are always context-dependent and require the physicians' prudence. What would be reasonable in an average US city may not be reasonable in a remote part of a developing country. And age matters insofar as the health of an eighty-year-old is more tenuous and attenuated, all else being equal, than that of a twenty-five-year-old.

We are not claiming that patients lose the authority to refuse medical interventions — even those interventions that have great promise for restoring health. If Mrs. Garcia had stated clearly that she was never to be intubated, period, her physicians should decline to intubate her as a matter of respect for the patient's authority to make such decisions prospectively; her decision-making authority can be respected, even if she has no autonomy to respect. The patient's authority is all the more in view if he or she has taken some legal step to give that refusal force and indicate that the decision is a considered one.

Because patients cannot anticipate every contingency, however, living wills are generally less useful than are DPOAHCs. Unlike living wills, DPOAHCs allow a patient to delegate authority for future decision-making to a person the patient trusts. Even if the objective is to secure decisions that the patient would have made if she were able to make them for herself, the DPOAHC is preferable insofar as the patient can have in-depth discussions with her authorized surrogate and give the surrogate the flexibility to fit a future decision to the complexity of the patient's story and the details of the specific clinical situation. In any case, if an advance directive does not unambiguously address the clinical question at stake, physicians are taught to use the second procedural mechanism: surrogate decision-makers.

Surrogate Decision-making

The physicians intubate Nora Garcia. After a rocky course of three days, she is taken off the ventilator. She is very weak but improving slowly. The next morning, she is found unresponsive in bed. An urgent CT scan of her head finds a large hemorrhagic stroke. The doctors go to Mrs. Garcia's three grown children, who have now gathered, in order to have an urgent family conference and decide what to do next.

When a patient is incapacitated, someone must have the authority to make medical decisions for her. It seems reasonable that such authority resides with the one to whom the patient has explicitly granted it if the patient has a durable power of attorney for healthcare or, in the absence of such explicit declaration, to those closest to the patient: her spouse, adult children, and so on. But what standard should these surrogate decision-makers use in exercising their authority on Mrs. Garcia's behalf?

With its singular emphasis on patient autonomy, the PSM has come to affirm what is called the *substituted judgment* standard. Out of respect for patient autonomy, physicians are taught to approach the legal surrogate or surrogates—in this case, Mrs. Garcia's children—to explain the situation accurately, including the options that are technically feasible, legal, and available, and to encourage the surrogates to make the choice that the patient would make if she were able to choose. The physician might say, "The question is not what you think is best or what we might think is best. The question is this: what would she have wanted?"

The substituted judgment standard has several problems. First, substituted judgment, in such cases, seems to sustain a façade of respecting autonomy that both hides and distracts clinicians and surrogates away from the actual question faced: all things considered, what is a fitting way to care for this patient? One cannot respect what does not exist, and Mrs. Garcia does not possess autonomy in her state. Rather, she is utterly dependent on those who would care for her. Moreover, to divine what she would have chosen if she could have chosen for herself is an exercise fraught with uncertainty. Researchers have found that close family members, including spouses, are notoriously inaccurate in predicting what their loved ones would want in prospective clinical situations.[6]

A final problem with the substituted judgment standard is that it divests physicians of a responsibility that they are obligated to exercise. Because of the subjectivity of what the patient would have chosen if she could have chosen for herself, the substituted judgment standard puts physicians in a passive role of merely giving information and options, deferring to the surrogates to make an informed choice. The physicians' primary aim as healthcare professionals, however, is not to find what the patient would choose if she could do so. Rather, the physicians' aim is to find a way to preserve and restore the health of the patient that still can be reasonably preserved or restored and to do so in a way that respects the patient's authority to give consent only to those proposals that fit her vocation.

Although the patient's authority has moved to surrogate decision-makers, the physicians ought not assume a passive posture. They should listen to and consider the surrogates' statements about the patient's vocation—how she lived, what her obligations are, what she loved, what they think she would encourage them to choose if she could—and, as we will see, the surrogates' statements about their own vocations. The physicians listen in order to propose courses of action that they believe align with the patient's health and vocation in light of this information.

The physicians should not by default encourage the family to "do everything." Indeed, in many cases the physicians can state, as the Hippocratic tradition suggested long ago,[7] that medicine has little left to offer other than solidarity and basic care. Health is a good that cannot be preserved forever, and in Mrs. Garcia's representative case, the patient's surrogates might reasonably focus on other goods. The primary point is that when a patient cannot exercise her authority to give consent for medical interventions, that authority shifts to the patient's surrogates, but the structure of the physician's discernment remains the same: the goal is to find a course of action that aligns with the physicians' orientation to the patient's health while remaining open to other basic human goods and the relevant truths about the patient's vocation.

Yet another question arises here: whose vocation is to guide the surrogate(s)' decision-making? The answer is that the surrogates' vocations now provide the relevant standard. Thus our view not only differs sharply from the substituted judgment standard but also differs somewhat from the *best-interest* standard. According to the latter, surrogates should judge and act in accordance with what is objectively best (often identified as in the "medical best interest") for the patient. That standard is superior to the substituted judgment standard insofar as it reflects the truth that surrogate decision-makers are charged to care for the ill and incapacitated patient, making the patient's welfare central to their consideration.

But surrogates have other concerns and other vocational commitments. They may have children or spouses who depend on them. They may have jobs to do and bills to pay. Surrogates can't abandon these. Accordingly, the terms discussed earlier—*extraordinary* and *ordinary* burdens and treatments—become apt for the surrogates' consideration. They are faced with options whose benefits and burdens bear not only on the patient but also on the surrogates themselves. Which interventions are ordinary and which are extraordinary now has to be determined in light of the surrogates' vocations—vocations that include but are not limited to obligations to care for the loved one in question.

Intention and Proportionality: A Case Study

Abe Anderson opts for chemotherapy, planning to receive an infusion biweekly for three months. Six weeks into this plan, repeat radiographic imaging reveals that his tumors have grown despite treatment. Meanwhile, he has lost thirty pounds and is starting to have severe abdominal and back pain. Vicodin no longer relieves the pain, and Abe's doctor recommends scheduled doses of morphine. Abe's wife worries about his being sedated and about addiction to opioids.

How can Abe's physician reasonably prescribe morphine in this case, when she knows that doing so likely will lead to her patient's physiological dependence on morphine? Once again, we must advert to the rule of double effect. Administering morphine has good effects—relief of pain—and bad effects: constipation, sedation, dependence, and more. What makes the physician's action reasonable, according to that rule, is that she intends only the good effects—in this case, the relief of Abe's health-diminishing pain—and that proportionality rests between the expected goods and harms. This judgment of proportionality is not a matter of looking for one choice that maximizes the net goods; no such choice can be known due to the goods' incommensurability. It is a matter of considering the gravity of the goods and harms at stake.

For example, if Mr. Anderson's pain were minor, the physician would have less reason to administer morphine. Proportionality also governs dosing: physicians need not be squeamish about giving adequate pain relief, but they are prevented from giving dosages that far exceed what one might reasonably expect to relieve Mr. Anderson's pain.

In this case, however, Abe's pain is serious. Given that he has relatively little time left to live, the risk of dependency does not seem as significant as it might otherwise. So it seems reasonable to prescribe him morphine to address his pain, provided that the side effects of constipation and sedation are acceptable to him.

> *Over the next two weeks, Abe Anderson grows steadily weaker and sleepier, often remaining in a state of somnolence. His wife wonders if the doctors are overmedicating him.*

Mrs. Anderson's question points to the difference the Way of Medicine makes. In the PSM, her concern prompts a question: what does Mr. Anderson really want, or what would he choose if he could choose for himself? If Abe's current experience suggests that the morphine dosing is not hitting the right balance, his doctors can adjust the medication according to his desires. In the PSM, whether the physicians are disposed to increase or decrease the dosing in this case depends entirely on the patient's wishes. Indeed, family members often ask that medication doses be increased to preclude any possibility of the patient's suffering.

The Way of Medicine, in contrast, returns once more to the norm of Mr. Anderson's health, with the rule of double effect helping the physicians stay on track. Is the morphine achieving the relief of health-diminishing pain, and is it doing so in a way that is proportionate to the adverse side effects? Can the former be achieved in a way that does not bring as much of the latter? These questions require the physicians' clinical judgment, which changes when circumstances change. For example, the effects of sedation that seemed minor when accepted as a consequence of relieving severe pain may seem more consequential when they are the consequence of moving from adequately relieved to completely relieved pain. Accepting some level of discomfort might be reasonable in order for Abe to maintain some degree of consciousness, if doing so allows him to interact with his family and to prepare himself for death. On the other hand, the sedation that was a heavy burden when it kept Mr. Anderson from putting his affairs in order may become a minor burden when he is actively dying.

Critically, Abe's physician rightly limits herself to those actions that are congruent with her commitment to her patient's health. She would be reticent, for example, to push the morphine dose high enough to render Mr. Anderson unconscious, even though by so doing she could prevent any further suffering. But she would also be reticent to watch her patient writhe in agony while abstemiously titrating up the dosing in tiny intervals out of concern for going too high. Finding the right practice here requires judgment, which is gained through long years of experience in pursuing patients' health while respecting the requirements of practical reason.

> *Nora Garcia's children were conflicted when her physicians asked them to decide whether she should be intubated or not. In the context of their uncertainty, the physicians intubated Mrs. Garcia. Three weeks later, she coughs when her airway is suctioned, but she still has not recovered enough to respond meaningfully to voice or touch. She receives ventilator support via a tracheostomy and nutrition via a feeding tube inserted through her abdominal wall. At this point, her three children together come to the physicians, saying, "We had hoped she would recover, but she has not. She would never have wanted to continue like this." The children ask that the ventilator be discontinued. "Just keep her comfortable," they say.*

In the PSM, the physician's obligations in regard to removing the ventilator are straightforward. The law allows life-sustaining technology to be discontinued; the duly appointed surrogates are requesting that it be discontinued; and, moreover, they are doing so according to the substituted judgment standard—they are making the request that they believe Mrs. Garcia would make if she were able. To make sure the surrogates' choice is informed, the physicians should tell the surrogates what they expect will happen as a result of discontinuing the ventilator, but then the physicians must do what is requested.

An additional issue arises: how to keep Mrs. Garcia comfortable when and after the ventilator is removed. Should narcotics and sedatives be given prospectively to reduce the chance that she will experience breathlessness and subsequent distress in the short time she is expected to live after life support is withdrawn? If so, what norms guide the dosing of such medications? Again, the answer is easy in the PSM: the norm is to minimize suffering and maximize quality of life according to the wishes of the patient or her surrogates. Therefore, after explaining to the family how the drugs work, the physicians are obligated to give a dosage that meets the family's expectations for their loved one's comfort. That dosage may be quite disproportionate to the discomfort the physicians expect their patient to experience if the surrogate decision-makers' primary concern is minimizing the possibility of any suffering.

Here the PSM and the Way of Medicine again overlap somewhat, despite their different starting points. In the Way of Medicine, the first question is how can removal of the ventilator be consistent with the physician's commitment to the patient's health? The second is how is removal of the ventilator consistent with the requirements of practical reason?

Mrs. Garcia's physicians are confident that she will die shortly after the ventilator is removed. How can anyone, much less a physician, remove the ventilator knowing that the patient will die as a result? Once more, guidance comes from the rule of double effect. The physician's commitment is to seek to preserve and restore his patient's health using reasonable means, insofar as the patient grants the physician the authority to do so. Keeping Mrs. Garcia on the ventilator provides at least a modicum of her health insofar as it maintains her life, and maintaining her life allows for further steps to be taken to improve her health, even if such steps do not hold much promise in her case. Thus keeping Mrs. Garcia on the ventilator can be reasonable as medicine.

But the ventilator's contribution to Mrs. Garcia's health, while real, is also relatively minor. In her case, use of the ventilator does not make possible further interventions to recover her lost health. Indeed, while medical technology can keep her alive indefinitely, little to no prospect remains for further healing. Moreover, the ventilator brings significant burdens: it is expensive; it requires Mrs. Garcia to stay in an intensive care unit; and it is relatively intrusive to her body, obstructing certain natural pathways of human interaction between her caregivers and her.

While Mrs. Garcia's physicians have some reason to maintain ventilator support, they should also respect the health-related limits of doing so, and the fact that her surrogates might reasonably judge that the burdens of continuing ventilator support are disproportionate to the benefits. Those surrogates can consistently treat Mrs. Garcia's life and health as goods while also judging that the ventilator should be removed in order to avoid the burdens associated with it—expense, intrusiveness, and so on. They can and should make that judgment in light of their own vocational commitments, which might include honoring what they believe their mother would have wanted—to end her days in the personal company of her loved ones rather than in the impersonal company of machines.

In choosing to discontinue the ventilator, neither the surrogates nor the physicians need to aim at the patient's death. The surrogates can choose to avoid certain burdens and to pursue a certain kind of human and personal environment for their remaining time with Mrs. Garcia, aware that death will likely be hastened as a side effect of seeking those benefits (including avoiding those burdens). The physicians can accommodate the surrogates' choice either because they share their intentions or if for some reason they disagree with the surrogates' judgment, because they intend to honor the surrogates' legitimate authority. In neither case do the physicians intend Mrs. Garcia's death either as a means or as an end. The surrogates and the physicians can act reasonably here in discontinuing the use of Mrs. Garcia's ventilator.

Of course, different circumstances would affect our judgment. Imagine, for example, that with two weeks more mechanical ventilation, Mrs. Garcia would likely return to the health she enjoyed before she fell ill. Then the burdens of mechanical ventilation for two weeks would not appear disproportionate to its anticipated benefits. The ventilator would be seen as ordinary treatment, and discontinuing it would be unethical. But even these judgments depend on considerations over which the surrogates have authority. The Way of Medicine respects that authority, allowing the physician to cooperate with an action that the physician would not choose herself.

Furthermore, what is true of the physicians relative to the surrogates is true of both relative to the patient. If Mrs. Garcia were to recover decisional capacity, she would have authority to ask that the ventilator be discontinued even if it was thought that only two weeks more of ventilation were needed to bridge her movement to a promising new treatment. That decision might be wrongful, and her family and physicians should voice their concerns, but the competent patient's authority to refuse medical interventions is almost absolute. Surrogates and physicians can intend to honor that authority while accepting as side effects the consequences of a patient's wrongful choice.

Surrogates' authority is more constrained than patients' authority. Traditionally, surrogates' decisions have been required to meet what has been called a *reasonable person standard*. If a surrogate makes a request that no reasonable person would choose (for example, removal of a ventilator right after a major surgery, before the patient has had a chance for anesthesia to wear off), the request will exceed the surrogates' authority and physicians may refuse it.

Let's now return to the question of Mrs. Garcia's comfort when the ventilator is withdrawn. The physicians' goals must remain tethered to the norm of the patient's health and subject to the questions of intention and proportionality. That the patient will die soon does not justify setting these considerations aside, though neither does the physicians' commitment to health mean that they must be tentative in administering medications to relieve breathlessness. Patients who die of respiratory failure often appear to experience profound distress from breathlessness, gasping for air as if drowning. Such a state is not one of health. Relieving such a state would seem to be an act required of healthcare professionals.

So a physician administers medication to mitigate breathlessness. Here we note a story from the clinical experience of one of the authors. Dr. Curlin was caring for a patient on a general medical service during training. The patient, an elderly woman, had suffered a devastating stroke, very much like the one Mrs. Garcia suffered, but instead of placing a tracheostomy, the family asked that the ventilator be withdrawn, recognizing that the patient would die. The patient was moved to a private room on the general medical floor, where her family could be present while the ventilator was withdrawn. When evaluating the patient, Dr. Curlin observed no spontaneous respirations and no response to painful stimuli. He asked the nurse to have a couple of doses of morphine available should the patient appear to be suffering breathlessness or distress as she died. After the ventilator was withdrawn, the patient did not breathe for more than a minute. Then she began to gasp. She grimaced, and sweat broke out on her brow. Her chest heaved, as if she was struggling to breathe but could not. Dr. Curlin called for the morphine to be administered, but in the five minutes it took for the nurse to access the IV and deliver the medication, the patient had died.

This was poor medicine. Dr. Curlin should have anticipated the possibility, even probability, that the patient would have a residual drive to breathe. Knowing that she would likely not be able to breathe sufficiently to survive, he should have given a dose of medication in advance that would have relieved her air hunger, and then had medicine available to be administered immediately, titrated to signs of such distress. Such an act would have been medicine truly in service of mercy. An important part of the physician's vocational commitment is to be concerned with patient health even in life's final moments, and the relief of breathlessness when a ventilator has been removed is a genuine manifestation of this commitment.

Poor medicine can also involve setting aside proportionality or embracing impermissible intentions. Physicians sometimes start a morphine infusion simply because a patient is expected to die, and then the infusion is titrated for no reason other than that the patient has not died yet. To give an example, palliative medicine colleagues of Dr. Curlin once were asked to see a patient in the ICU who had not recovered from a major surgery. The family asked that life-sustaining technology be withdrawn. The palliative medicine team left recommendations for medication to relieve distress, with dosing proportionate to what they expected would be needed. They returned hours later to find the patient profoundly sedated on doses of narcotics and sedatives much higher than they had recommended. When they asked about such high dosing, the surgical team said that the family was distressed that it was taking so long for the patient to die. This case and others like it demonstrate physicians detaching from the norm of the patient's health, instead beginning to aim at the patient's death. When medication dosing becomes disproportionate to what is needed to relieve disabling symptoms, something has gone wrong.

Unfortunately, the PSM conditions physicians to ignore, or even to welcome, these departures from proportionality and an orientation to the patient's health. After all, the point of the PSM is to relieve, using the tools at hand, the conditions that the patient or her surrogate suffers. When being alive comes to be experienced as a burden, the physician's tools can quickly become death-dealing, opening the patient up to the expanding domain of so-called last-resort options.

CHAPTER NINE

Last-Resort Options

In this chapter we meet patients who are not only at the end of life but seemingly at the end of hope. What should physicians do when patients are dying and have nothing left to look forward to except pain and misery? We have already established that physicians have good reasons to treat pain and other symptoms effectively, and at times to accept substantial side effects of such treatment, including even the effect of hastening death. But some patients want more. They want to die on their own terms, not wait for their illnesses to bring about their death in unwanted ways. In particular, they experience a state of profound and irreversible debility and dependence as one that is worse than being dead. What can be done for such patients?

In the provider of services model (PSM), physicians facing such cases are urged to consider what their proponents call "last-resort options" for palliative care. These include encouraging the patient to voluntarily stop eating and drinking, administering palliative sedation to unconsciousness, and, most prominently, offering assisted suicide and euthanasia. What makes all of these practices controversial is the question of intention: is the patient's death intended in these practices? If so, on the Way of Medicine, such practices are ruled out from the start.

Not so under the PSM. Rather, clinicians pursue the goals of minimizing suffering and maximizing quality of life without any absolute prohibitions, not even the prohibition against killing one's patient. At the time of this writing, assisted suicide and euthanasia remain illegal in most US jurisdictions; for the moment, in most jurisdictions such practices are not in the universe of options that physicians must offer patients. But when that changes—as it has changed in several US states, all of Canada, and several European nations—the PSM not only permits assisted suicide and euthanasia; it can require physicians to accommodate patients' requests for these options, at least by referring them to someone who will provide them. The PSM approach centers on its commitment to use medical technologies to bring about *well-being*. After all, how can a patient be said to have well-being if he lives when he wants to die, particularly when he obviously suffers a degraded and steadily diminishing quality of life?

When the goal of medicine shifts from helping patients who are dying to helping patients to die, practices that hasten death no longer seem like last-resort options. Indeed, such practices seem to follow ineluctably from making the relief of suffering—an alternate formulation of *well-being*—medicine's first principle. Medicine aims to minimize suffering and maximize quality of life according to the patient's judgment and values. The patient is suffering and experiences a poor quality of life. The clinician has the tools to make the suffering go away by making the condition of being alive and conscious—which makes suffering possible—go away. Although intentionally bringing about the patient's death would seem to contradict the goal of preserving and restoring health, medicine is no longer constrained by such goals. Therefore, the clinician may, and is perhaps morally obligated to, offer the patient various means by which the patient can bring about the end of his life.

Before we get too far ahead of ourselves in discussing "last-resort options," let's consider cases that involve continuing or withdrawing nutrition and hydration. How would the Way of Medicine approach these practices?

ARTIFICIAL NUTRITION AND HYDRATION

Nora Garcia is moved to a private room for her use of the ventilator to be discontinued. When that is done, despite the physicians' expectations, Mrs. Garcia breathes on her own, so a few days after

*that she is moved to a long-term nursing facility. Six weeks later
she has developed a bedsore but is otherwise clinically stable. Her
family now asks that tube feeding be discontinued.*

The laws of most nations allow tube feeding, or artificial nutrition
and hydration (ANH) to be discontinued at the request of a patient or
the patient's surrogates. The reasonable-person standard applies to the
latter, but that standard would allow physicians to remove the feeding
tube in Mrs. Garcia's case, just as many otherwise reasonable persons
elect to discontinue tube feeding in similar cases.

According to the PSM, the physician's obligation here is straightforward: inform the surrogates of what can be expected with continuing or discontinuing the tube feedings, ask them to imagine what Mrs.
Garcia would choose if she could, and then accommodate the surrogates' choice. In such situations, surrogates and clinicians often talk
about choosing quality of life and comfort over degradation and suffering. They might talk about allowing the patient to die with dignity.
The application of such concepts, along with the four principles guiding the practice of medicine (autonomy, beneficence, nonmaleficence,
and justice), tends to hinge on the ideal of authentic choice: choosing
what the patient would have chosen if she were able.

Thus, for example, if the surrogates say that Mrs. Garcia would
never have wanted to live like this, they or Mrs. Garcia's physicians
might conclude that continuing the tube feeding violates the duty not
to harm because it forces her to endure a degraded condition, or poor
quality of life. If, alternatively, the surrogates decide that the patient
would have chosen to continue the tube feeding (believing, perhaps,
"She would have wanted everything done"), discontinuing the feeding
would seem to violate the same duty not to harm, or at least fail to fulfill the principle of beneficence by withholding something from which
the patient benefits. Again, everything turns on what the patient would
have wanted.

Of course, when the patient clearly has refused ANH prospectively, or at present still has the capacity to refuse, the case is even
clearer: the physicians must accommodate the refusal. But what is
notable, and notably different from the Way of Medicine, is just what

surrogates and clinicians are respecting when accommodating such refusals. If the patient refuses nutrition and hydration in order to die, then proponents of the PSM generally suggest that the decision itself is to be honored out of respect for patient autonomy. The thinking here is straightforward: the patient decides whether his life is worth living. If he decides it is not, that settles the question of what should be done, despite what seems a clearly suicidal intention.

By contrast, the Way of Medicine holds that life is always a good, and the complex good of life and health is the object of medical commitment. Accordingly, a patient cannot reasonably refuse artificial nutrition and hydration—whether by advance directive or in the moment—if his goal in doing so is to bring about his death. Likewise, a clinician or surrogate who cooperates in that decision in order to bring about the patient's death is doing something wrong—contrary both to practical reason and to the norms of medicine.

Having said that, cooperation with the patient's request is not entirely ruled out. While the Way of Medicine does not ask clinicians to respect an unreasonable choice, it does ask them to respect patients' authority to make such a choice. Thus, doctors are not to refuse a patient's request to discontinue ANH, even if the patient's choice is unreasonable. The doctors cooperate in order to honor the patient's legitimate authority, however, not to bring about the patient's death.

Moreover, patients can refuse ANH uprightly. A patient might, for example, decide in advance not to ask certain forms of care of their future caregivers, out of concern for those caregivers. Or, sensitive to the limits both of health and of medicine, the very elderly might ask not to be encumbered with tubes when their time is already short. Both of these reasons for setting limits to medical interventions are legitimate, and generally where the possibility of an upright refusal exists, the patient's legitimate exercise of authority is to be respected even if one strongly suspects that that authority is being misused in a particular case.

Thus, when it comes to refusing artificial nutrition and hydration, the Way of Medicine overlaps with the PSM in acknowledging a patient's authority to refuse medical interventions, including ANH, and it contradicts the PSM in rejecting suicide and any intentional cooperation with it.

Mrs. Garcia's case differs from the cases just described, however, insofar as she did not request prospectively that she not receive artificial nutrition and hydration. What should the physicians do? They and Mrs. Garcia's surrogates should deliberate in the same way that they deliberated about removing the ventilator. The rule of double effect still applies, though among proponents of the Way of Medicine, some disagree with the notion that tube feeding in a case like Mrs. Garcia's can reasonably be considered to have a burden that is disproportionate to the benefits it provides. Further, some worry that under the pretense of removing a burdensome intervention, those who want to discontinue ANH for Mrs. Garcia are actually making the removal a means of bringing about her death.

Recall that the tube feeding may be discontinued if it is disproportionately burdensome—that is, extraordinary. This presupposes that real benefits accrue to continued feeding, for if feeding becomes strictly futile (e.g., if the patient develops a bowel obstruction), it would be unreasonable for physicians to even offer to continue it. But in Mrs. Garcia's case ANH helps to maintain her life and health (if there is no life, there is no health, and vice versa). These are genuine goods for all human beings, and Mrs. Garcia remains a human being.

Of course, some people object that Mrs. Garcia's life and health are of value only insofar as they make it possible for Mrs. Garcia to pursue other goods. If that is true, ANH is no benefit to her, because her life and health are of no further instrumental value. This claim is incompatible with the requirements of practical reason, however, for all the basic goods are intrinsically good for all human beings. It is also incompatible with a straightforward inference from a basic claim. If we consider ourselves as having intrinsic value and acknowledge that we are living animal organisms, our biological lives must be of intrinsic value, for that which constitutes the existence of a being with intrinsic value must itself have intrinsic value. So we take this objection to be misconceived: Mrs. Garcia's life and health remains good in itself, even if she can realize that good only to a minimal degree.

Feeding Mrs. Garcia also realizes the good of solidarity—a form of friendship, of being humanly and personally connected to another, willing his or her good for its own sake, and engaging in care for them when they are in need. Some actions clearly would violate such solidarity: dressing Mrs. Garcia up like a clown for the amusement of others, violating her physical integrity, and the like. Caring for her—and feeding is a primordial form of caring—realizes the good of friendship even if Mrs. Garcia does not consciously experience it.[1]

Does ANH bring burdens? Yes. Tube feeding brings costs as well as risks of infection, aspiration, and other clinical complications. Whether Mrs. Garcia suffers as a result of her feeding tubes is hard to say. The burdens ANH imposes on her seem relatively light, if not trivial. However, some patients who are not in Mrs. Garcia's circumstances face further burdens. Patients with Alzheimer's disease, for example, are sometimes distressed by feeding tubes and tear them out; preventing their doing so can require chemical or physical restraints, which impose significant burdens of their own. Such burdens could warrant withdrawing the tubes to avoid these (disproportionate) burdens. Likewise, if a patient is actively dying or is otherwise unable to assimilate nutrition, the benefits of feeding will not be proportionate to the burdens, and feeding may be discontinued. But in Mrs. Garcia's case, it seems less clear that continuing ANH brings disproportionate burdens.

ANH should not be discontinued with the intention of bringing about Mrs. Garcia's death, and this principle raises a particular difficulty for one response to the question of proportionality. In that response, the surrogates or physicians might note that the burdens of care for Mrs. Garcia are quite significant: she is in a nursing facility, which is expensive, and watching and visiting her in this state is emotionally and physically taxing for her family, while her wound care is tedious for the nurses. Surely these burdens, one might argue, are disproportionate to the minor benefit of continued life in a state of radically diminished health.

The practical reasoning advocated in the Way of Medicine looks to the burdens and benefits of a particular intervention to ask whether there is proportionality or disproportionality between the good and bad effects of that intervention. But here, for Mrs. Garcia, the intervention in question is tube feeding. We have identified the benefits (life and health) and burdens (cost, risk of infection) of that intervention. Discontinuing tube feeding removes, in itself, precisely those burdens; it does not, as such, remove the overall costs of hospital care or the overall emotional and physical burdens of caring for Mrs. Garcia. What removes *those* burdens is Mrs. Garcia's death. So the choice to withdraw ANH in order to end those burdens seems to involve intending Mrs. Garcia's death. Such a choice is impermissible on the Way of Medicine.

Deliberating reasonably in this case requires focusing on the benefits and burdens of the tube feeding itself. If the benefits of ANH are proportionate to the burdens of ANH, the burdens should be accepted. That said, it remains the case that one of us (Tollefsen) thinks that Mrs. Garcia should certainly be fed in this case (though she might be brought home if that would alleviate the other burdens of her care), while the other (Curlin) believes that the vocational shape of Mrs. Garcia's life may in some cases be better honored by keeping her as free from technological interventions, including feeding tubes, as possible. So Curlin believes one might reasonably judge that ANH, in Mrs. Garcia's case, no longer promises benefits proportionate to the burdens of ANH itself (however minor those appear to be). Disagreement is not impossible for those committed to the Way of Medicine.

We return now to the last-resort options, the first of which also involves nutrition and hydration.

Last-Resort Options

Abe Anderson is declining. His oncologists stop his chemotherapy. He elects to receive hospice care at home. His pain worsens, requiring steadily increasing doses of morphine. He manages to stay awake most of the time. The hospice physician comes to see him at home a few weeks later. In their conversation, Mr. Anderson notes, "I don't want to languish, doc. I want to go out on my own terms. What can I do if I don't want to go on any longer?"

Voluntary Cessation of Eating

Abe's question invites his physician to offer last-resort options. The first such option is for Abe to voluntarily stop eating (and/or drinking). In that case, Abe's remaining days would be few, and with adequate morphine those days could be made relatively painless. But as we already noted, this choice includes a lethal intention: Abe would forgo nutrition and hydration in order to hasten his death, an intention ruled out by the demands of practical reason. The Way of Medicine likewise rules out recommending or suggesting such an approach, even if it would be wrong to force nutrition and hydration on a patient who had given up on eating. So the physician should not offer Abe the opportunity to starve himself to death, as if that were a legitimate medical option.

This case must be distinguished from an otherwise similar scenario. Patients who are dying often begin to withdraw from food and water. As we have noted, in the final days of a terminal illness, nutrition often cannot be assimilated, but even somewhat before this point, patients with advanced illness can find themselves with no desire to eat and even with revulsion at the thought of food. Turning away from food under such circumstances does not seem to us a suicidal choice, but rather a choice to avoid something that no longer seems enjoyable or meaningful in the way it once did. If death is hastened by this choice, that is a proportionate and morally permissible side effect.

Sedation to Unconsciousness

A second "last resort option" would be to sedate Abe so that he lives out his last days free of any conscious suffering. In what has come to be called *palliative sedation to unconsciousness*, formerly known as *terminal sedation*,[2] physicians intentionally sedate patients to the point of unconsciousness and keep them unconscious until they die. This differs from what is called *proportionate palliative sedation*, in which sedatives are used for the purpose of relieving anxiety, agitation, breathlessness, or other symptoms, and diminished consciousness is foreseen as a side effect but not intended.

We have written at length elsewhere about the ethics of palliative sedation,[3] but we first want to emphasize that the Way of Medicine supports proportionate palliative sedation. As long as the clinician aims only to relieve health-diminishing symptoms and has proportionate reason to accept unconsciousness as a side effect (thus satisfying the rule of double effect), the sedation is morally permissible, even in cases in which it is expected that sedation will continue until the patient dies. Indeed, physicians cannot act to relieve health-diminishing symptoms except by accepting some level of sedation as a side effect of their efforts. Almost all of the medications used to relieve pain and other symptoms cause sedation as a side effect. This is true of narcotics, of course, but also of medications to relieve anxiety, seizures, delirium, nausea, and itching. To treat sedation as a side effect aligns with the fact that patients and their families generally do not want their sensoriums clouded or their capacities to think, talk, and pursue the goods available to them blunted, but most will accept these losses if they are side effects of efforts to relieve disabling symptoms, particularly at the end of life.

We also note that proportionate palliative sedation can relieve disabling and distressing symptoms in nearly all if not all clinical circumstances. In his book *Dying Well: Peace and Possibilities at the End of Life*, Ira Byock, a seasoned hospice physician, describes a case in which he came finally to intentionally sedate a dying patient to unconsciousness because the patient's severe pain had proven refractory to every other treatment modality.[4] Those who advocate for sedation to unconsciousness as a form of physician aid-in-dying often invoke cases like the one Dr. Byock described, just as advocates for physician-assisted suicide and euthanasia invoke cases of excruciating and untreatable pain. But these appeals are red herrings. Dr. Byock noted that the case he described was the only such case he had experienced in more than fifteen years of caring for dying patients.[5] One of the authors of this book (Curlin) has practiced hospice and palliative medicine for more than ten years and has never encountered a patient whose pain or other disabling symptoms could not be relieved under the norms of proportionate palliative sedation. Last-resort options in general, and palliative sedation to unconsciousness in particular, are used much more commonly to relieve a type of suffering that is quite distinct from the pain experienced by Dr. Byock's patient. They are used to relieve *existential suffering*.

Sedation to unconsciousness to relieve existential suffering contradicts the norms of the Way of Medicine. Consider first the character of existential suffering, and then how the capacity for wakefulness relates to human health. Suffering is, to some extent, inevitable in dying, for dying is in its nature an evil—not a moral evil, but a privation of something always and everywhere good: namely, human life and, more specifically, the life of a person. While death is not to be feared above all things, and while we believe that hope in eternal life should accompany death, nevertheless, death is not good, and *suffering itself is the experience of that which is not as it should be*.[6] So the experience of illness and the prospect of imminent death usually bring suffering, whether or not the patient experiences pain or other symptoms. Pain and other symptoms heighten suffering in their direct, noxious effects on conscious experience and also insofar as they disrupt our ability to do what humans otherwise do when they are healthy. Moreover, patients who are dying often experience alienation from themselves, their friends and family, and even God. All of these bring suffering.

Existential suffering is the cognitive awareness of that which is not as it should be. At the end of life, a patient may experience such suffering through revulsion at the threat of death, regret at missed opportunities and botched choices, sorrow over failed or ruptured relationships, or fear of the divine. These are real problems and real forms of suffering. As such, they require choices, attempts to maintain or restore what harmony is possible at the end of life: acceptance of death, repentance of sin, reconciliation with loved ones, and peace with God.

Sedation to unconsciousness cuts short all of these possible responses to existential suffering. While perhaps not a choice for death as such, it is a choice for a kind of *moral* death, putting oneself existentially out of reach of these and all other possibilities. Such possibilities can be dramatic: those who have read the novel *Brideshead Revisited* (or seen the miniseries) can call to mind Lord Marchmain's literal deathbed conversion, which restored him both to his religion and, in various ways, to his family.[7] Thus he was restored to the forms of harmony and integrity available to him even at the very end of life. But integrity and harmony (with reality, with one's self, with others, with God) are basic goods, and the opportunity to pursue them should not be discarded without exceptionally strong reason. Sedation to unconsciousness to avoid existential suffering, rather than to treat refractory and crippling pain or other symptoms, thus seems to us incompatible with being fully open to human goods.

Consider now how the capacity for wakefulness relates to human health. Making a patient permanently unconscious diminishes the patient's health; that seems an uncontroversial point insofar as the capacity for wakefulness is an expression of health. Here we must distinguish the state of suppressed consciousness from the state of sleep, in which the individual is capable of arousal. We also must distinguish keeping a person unconscious until he dies from sedating him temporarily, as physicians often do as part of their efforts (e.g., surgery) to preserve or restore health. It seems that in most cases, and certainly in the case of existential suffering, physicians who intentionally and permanently sedate patients to unconsciousness thereby contradict the purposes of medicine.

In a very rare case, however, palliative sedation to unconsciousness would be permissible. In that scenario, the patient would suffer, or be expected to imminently suffer, such a severe form of altered—diseased, unhealthy, disabling—consciousness that it would make sense to cut off this unhealthy consciousness in the same way it makes sense sometimes to cut off a severely diseased (say, gangrenous) limb. In such a case, we can say that the patient's health is diminished by virtue of losing consciousness or a limb, but his health is less diminished without the consciousness or the limb than with it. A part can be sacrificed for the health of a whole. Put differently, to the extent that suppressing consciousness allows the organism to relax from a state of high physical and psychic stress, such unconsciousness might be an expression of health, albeit of a radically diminished sort. Such sedation could continue until death if a return to consciousness is expected to bring a return to high levels of distress refractory to proportionate palliative sedation.

While such cases are exceedingly rare, Dr. Byock's patient may have met this criterion, and in Dr. Curlin's experience, some cases of agitated delirium (often called *terminal delirium*) at the end of life also may meet this criterion. Still, we caution against the tendency to amputate consciousness too readily, even in such cases. That tendency seems driven by pressures and temptations—since patients who are unconscious require less of the physician's attention—to make the appearance of suffering go away.[8]

Physician-Assisted Suicide and Voluntary Euthanasia

In the final last-resort options, a physician might prescribe a lethal dose of some medication in order to help Abe take his own life (*physician-assisted suicide*) or, alternatively, perhaps because Abe is too weak to do so himself, the physician might administer the lethal dose himself (*voluntary euthanasia*). We refer to both of these options as *physician aid-in-dying*.

Let us begin our discussion of physician-assisted suicide and voluntary euthanasia not with our fictional case studies involving Mr. Anderson or Mrs. Garcia but with a real case, one of the most influential in making the public argument for physician aid-in-dying in our time.

Brittany Maynard was diagnosed with brain cancer in January 2014; she was twenty-nine years old. In the remaining eight months of her life, she became a prominent public advocate for legalization of physician-assisted suicide. She moved from California to Oregon and, according to a plan she had specified in advance, died on November 1 of that year after ingesting a lethal physician-prescribed drug cocktail. Unquestionably, as a young, attractive, and tragic face of the right-to-die movement, Ms. Maynard, as Arthur Caplan put it, "shifted the optics of the debate."[9]

Ms. Maynard's story illustrates a pattern: those who seek physician aid-in-dying are rarely driven by the direct experience of refractory pain or other symptoms.[10] At the time she committed suicide, Ms. Maynard was not experiencing symptoms beyond the reach of conventional palliative medicine, nor are such symptoms expected from a brain tumor. Rather, as she said, she chose to end her life on her own terms in order to avoid the prospect of further debility and decline, in which she might "suffer personality changes and verbal, cognitive and motor loss of virtually any kind."[11]

Ms. Maynard's desire to avoid debility and dependence reflects the pattern found in official reports from Oregon and Washington State, where nine out of ten patients requesting assisted suicide have reported being concerned about "losing autonomy" (91.5 percent) and being "less able to engage in activities making life enjoyable" (88.7 percent).[12]

The problem to which assisted suicide and euthanasia pose solutions, then, is not uncontrolled pain. In Oregon, only one in four patients (24.7 percent) have reported even "concern about" inadequate pain control,[13] and at no time in history have physicians and patients had greater access to effective tools for treating pain and other distressing symptoms, tools that can be deployed aggressively under ethical norms that have guided medicine for ages.

Rather, the problem to which aid-in-dying poses a solution is loss of control—the desire to sustain self-determination and autonomy in the face of debilitating illness. In a piece in the *Journal of the American Medical Association*, Dr. Timothy Quill and colleagues wrote, "Patients with serious illness wish to have control over their own bodies, their own lives, and concern about future physical and psychosocial distress."[14] Brittany Maynard put the point bluntly in her online manifesto: "I want to die on my own terms." Seen in this light, the movement toward physician aid-in-dying is the culmination of the PSM approach to medicine and medical ethics.

Ms. Maynard then added, "My question is who has the right to tell me that I don't deserve this choice?" That is a powerful question in our day. The former Hemlock Society is now called "Compassion and *Choices*" (emphasis ours).[15] The California law legalizing assisted suicide was called the End of Life *Option* Act (again, our emphasis).[16] When Governor Jerry Brown signed it, he said he did not know if he would avail himself of assisted suicide, but "I wouldn't deny that right to others."[17] Choice looms large.

But what kind of choice is Ms. Maynard and others like her being denied if physicians refuse to hasten their deaths? Ms. Maynard already had the right to refuse life-sustaining treatment. She had the right to proportionate palliation of her symptoms even if death were hastened as a side effect. She had the means and capacity to cause her death by numerous methods that do not involve physicians and that are equally if not more efficient and effective than ingesting an overdose of pharmaceuticals. Why is it so essential that she and others have physicians, in particular, cooperate in helping them kill themselves?

That physicians are being asked, or even required, to cooperate shows that "the right to choose" is, as the late Robert Burt noted, "radically incomplete as a justification for physician assisted suicide."[18] The right to choose has been transformed into a positive entitlement to have others help bring about what has been chosen—and not just any others, but medical professionals specifically. The physician aid-in-dying movement portends large-scale changes for the medical profession that will mark the definitive end of the Way of Medicine and the advent of a more authoritarian form of the PSM.

We discuss the PSM's exclusivist and authoritarian tendencies in chapter 10. Here we consider three questions that are central to evaluating the proposals for physician aid-in-dying. First, and most generally, how do the requirements of practical reason bear upon the practice of physician aid-in-dying? Second, how is physician aid-in dying related to the ends of medicine? And third, what will physician aid-in-dying do to patient trust?

The Requirements of Practical Reason and Killing at the End of Life

Practical reason's judgment on the question of physician aid-in-dying is in one sense quite straightforward. All the suggested forms of this practice, including physician-assisted suicide and voluntary euthanasia, involve intentional killing: the patient's death is the means to relieve her suffering or is the satisfaction of her desire to maintain control. But it is always wrong to intend the death of an innocent person. So one may not reasonably kill oneself, kill another, or help another to kill him- or herself. So far, then, the various forms of aid-in-dying seem little different morally from elective abortion.

But killing at the end of life differs from abortion in an important way. No abortion ever takes place with the consent of the unborn child, so except in vital conflict cases, such killing not only violates the moral norm that basic goods are not to be intentionally damaged or destroyed, but also the norm of fairness. (As our discussion of Judith Jarvis Thomson showed, the latter norm is usually violated even when the former norm is not.) In contrast—and the aid-in-dying movement makes much of this fact—those who seek physician assistance in death generally actively want and choose to die. While physician aid-in-dying clearly violates the norm against intentional killing, physician aid-in-dying for competent adults does not obviously violate the norm requiring fairness.

As a matter of clinical ethics, the norm requiring fairness is irrelevant insofar as killing the innocent is always wrong, and no morally upright physician or patient would participate in such killing. But fairness is a central part of justice, and justice is the paradigmatic social virtue. Political states and professional institutions are structured around the demands of justice. Even though an act might be morally wrong, if it is not a matter of injustice, the state is unlikely to show much concern. People arguing that the state and the medical profession should forbid physician aid-in-dying make a stronger case if they show the practice to be not only wrong but substantively unjust.

We believe this challenge can be met. Legalizing physician aid-in-dying is rightly a matter of political concern and concern for the medical profession, especially if it threatens to reshape medical practice in ways that portend harms to many unconsenting patients. Insofar as physician aid-in-dying poses such a threat, strong reasons persist to maintain vigorous legal and professional restrictions on the practice and to refuse to give physicians a right that no other citizen possesses: the right to intentionally cause the death of an innocent person.

The End of Medicine and Aid-in-Dying

The Way of Medicine also returns a quick answer to the question of physician aid-in-dying. The end of medicine is health, and the physician professes to seek health in patients. Physician-assisted suicide and voluntary euthanasia involve actions that intend the death of the patient, the first by means of cooperation with the patient's suicidal intention, the second by a direct action of the physician intended to end the patient's life. Few acts seem more distinctly contrary to the end and the vocational commitment of medicine, and for this reason alone, they have no place in the profession. Nor should physicians be expected, much less required, to aid or facilitate such actions, even by providing referrals.

For a profession in good order, this point would suffice. But the question remains: how are concerns of justice and fairness implicated

here? To address this question, we turn to a further, deeply related, objection to physician aid-in-dying: these practices threaten to erode
trust and trustworthiness—central virtues of the physician-patient
relationship, without which the profession cannot long continue.

Trust

Robert Burt, quoted earlier, also noted, "The confident assertion of the
self-determination right leaves unacknowledged and unanswered a
crucial background question: who can be trusted to care for me when
I am too vulnerable and fearful to care for myself?"[19]

His point is well taken. For every Abe Anderson and Brittany
Maynard who wants a physician to help them end their lives, physicians are called to care for numerous other radically diminished patients who, along with their families, count on physicians to care for
them, seeking to preserve and restore the health that remains insofar
as reasonably possible. An example from Curlin's practice makes the
point:

> Dr. Curlin was asked to see a patient in the emergency room.[20] The
> patient, Mr. Roberts, had advanced dementia; he had not spoken
> in three years. He was brought to the hospital by his brother and
> his niece, who for several years had cared for him at home. The
> emergency physician's initial evaluation made clear that Mr. Rob-
> erts had a serious pneumonia and was beginning to suffer septic
> shock and respiratory failure. After Dr. Curlin spoke briefly with
> Mr. Roberts's family members, they agreed with his proposal to
> give the patient antibiotics, oxygen, and other supportive therapy
> but to forgo mechanical ventilation, even if Mr. Roberts came to
> the point of not being able to breathe on his own. Dr. Curlin then
> asked the patient's brother and niece if they had ever considered
> hospice care for Mr. Roberts. Both shook their heads and said ada-
> mantly, "We are not interested in hospice." "Why is that?" Dr.
> Curlin asked. They responded that what they had seen indicated
> that hospice too often forgoes any effort to provide medical care for
> patients, instead focusing only on giving potent drugs like morphine
> and sedatives, and thereby hastening patients' death.

Mr. Roberts's family members' concern is one that Dr. Curlin has heard voiced by numerous other patients and family members in Durham, North Carolina, and on the South Side of Chicago, and it highlights a question that physicians must consider: with respect to physician aid-in-dying, which of the following should physicians care about most: maintaining the trust of those who, like Mr. Roberts and his family, already experience the debility, dependence, and suffering that advanced illness brings or empowering those who, like Brittany Maynard, seek through assisted suicide to avoid such debility, dependence, and suffering?

That was not a rhetorical question for Mr. Roberts's family. Indeed, like too many others, they had come to the conclusion that some physicians who wield the tools of palliative medicine are not to be trusted because such physicians have so prioritized relieving suffering that they fail to do what patients count on physicians to do: use reasonable means to preserve the health and lives of the patients. How much less likely would Mr. Roberts's family be to entrust him to a physician or group of physicians that is in the habit of practicing assisted suicide or euthanasia or encouraging people to stop eating or to stop feeding their loved ones? We doubt their worries would be assuaged upon hearing that the physicians do so "only for those who choose" these options.

Physicians cannot practice hastening or causing the deaths of their patients without undermining the trust on which the practice of medicine depends. This insight is not new. Physicians who care for patients with advanced illness have long known that everyone will at times be tempted to do away with suffering by doing away with the patient. To militate against that temptation, physicians have for more than two millennia sworn in the Hippocratic Oath, "I will neither give a deadly drug to anybody who asks for it, nor will I make a suggestion to this effect."[21] The American Medical Association has maintained since its founding, "Physician assisted suicide is fundamentally inconsistent with the physician's professional role."[22] The World Medical Association has opposed assisted suicide and euthanasia since the association was formed and issued the Declaration of Geneva just after the Second World War. Indeed, insofar as physicians enjoy the trust of patients made vulnerable by illness, it is because, since Hippocrates, at least, they have maintained solidarity with those who are sick and disabled, seeking only to heal and refusing to use their skills and powers to do harm. That is why physicians have refused to participate in capital punishment, to be active combatants, or to help patients commit suicide.

Importantly, this boundary against intentionally causing a patient's death not only gives patients a reason to trust physicians but also gives physicians the freedom they need to do their work. For example, Dr. Curlin was able to tell Mr. Roberts's family members that as a physician he is committed to *never* hasten or cause a patient's death intentionally. This boundary creates a space in which he and other physicians can act decisively to palliate distressing symptoms—for example, by using morphine to alleviate the apparent breathlessness that Mr. Roberts was experiencing or sedatives to relieve a state of restlessness and agitation in Abe Anderson. Without this boundary, Mr. Roberts's family has good reasons to worry that the morphine that leads to sedation is dosed not in proportion to the pain or breathlessness of their loved one but in an effort to hurry along the dying process.

To return to the question we posed above: which should be most important to physicians—maintaining the trust of those who, like Mr. Roberts and his family, already experience the debility, dependence, and suffering that advanced illness brings or empowering those who, like Brittany Maynard, seek through physician aid-in-dying to avoid such debility, dependence, and suffering? The witness of physicians and patients through the centuries and into the present has affirmed that we cannot have it both ways. But the question is central to determining the practice of medicine into the future.

At the heart of medicine is solidarity with those who are diminished in health, disabled in body, and therefore most dependent on trustworthy professionals devoted to their care. Physicians maintain solidarity with those who, to borrow Ms. Maynard's terms, suffer "verbal, cognitive and motor loss of virtually [every] kind," whether from developmental disabilities, traumatic injuries, dementia, or other debilitating chronic conditions. The countless patients who live with such conditions display a truth that Brittany Maynard could not see and that those suffering advanced illness may struggle to keep in view: debility and dependence do not render lives not worth living; human dignity does not require living or dying on one's own terms.

In a culture that emphasizes success and productivity, youthfulness and beauty, autonomy and control, such trust becomes obscured. The public images of Ms. Maynard made it conspicuously obvious that she possessed all of those when her disease struck, and her statements made it clear that she saw a condition in which these were lost as one worse than death. Not incidentally, those who advocate for and avail themselves of assisted suicide are overwhelmingly white, well-off, and accustomed to being able-bodied. According to official reports, of the 1,083 people who died in Oregon by assisted suicide prior to January 19, 2018, only 1 was African American (statistically, one would have expected at least 20, as 2.1 percent of Oregon's population is African American, according to the US Census).[23] In Washington State's March 2018 report, fewer than 4 percent of deaths by assisted suicide (from 2015 to 2017) were nonwhites, whereas 20 percent of the population was nonwhite.[24] Mr. Roberts's family, like most of Dr. Curlin's patients in Chicago and Durham, was African American. A population that already has experienced itself as vulnerable is more likely to see the practice of physician aid-in-dying not as a boon but as a threat.[25]

If "verbal, cognitive, and motor loss" renders life not worth living, you might think that disability groups would welcome physicians hastening or causing the deaths of those who so choose. But the opposite is the case. Disability groups overwhelmingly oppose assisted death. The prominent advocacy group Not Dead Yet speaks for many in arguing that "it cannot be seriously maintained" that legalization of assisted suicide will not lead to "inappropriate pressures from family or society" for people to end their lives. The group contends that "assisted suicide laws ensure legal immunity for physicians who already devalue the lives of older and disabled people and have significant economic incentives to at least agree with their suicides, if not encourage them, or worse."[26]

To summarize, under the approach we propose, assisted death is impermissible, first because it is never reasonable for anyone to kill the innocent or to help the innocent kill themselves. Assisted death is impermissible for physicians a fortiori, because killing contradicts the very nature of the practice of medicine and its orientation to the patient's health. If anyone is to help people take their lives, let it not be physicians. But even if these time-tested reasons have lost their grasp on our moral imaginations, it should be clear that it is unjust to purchase yet another choice for those accustomed to living life on their own terms at the cost of betraying physicians' distinctive solidarity with, and thereby undermining the trust of, those who live under the terms of illness and disability that they have not chosen, but with respect to which they should be able to count on physicians' care.

The question of trust points to the importance—not just for the medical profession, but also for society and law—of maintaining with strictest fidelity the norm against permitting doctors intentionally to kill their patients. The profession of medicine is socially of great value: it ensures that the good of those whose health is compromised will be pursued based on the solidarity of the healer and the patient. But that relationship remains unequal, and that inequality contributes to the patient's vulnerability. Clinical ethicist Richard Zaner has gone so far as to wonder what keeps physicians from acting like Plato's Gyges. When Gyges discovered a ring that made him invisible, he immediately killed the king and seduced his wife, taking advantage of his power in the assurance that he would not be caught.[27]

Zaner points to the importance of trust as a constitutive virtue for the medical profession, one without which there simply would be no such profession. Given the deep and abiding importance of medicine— we will *all* be sick, we will *all* be vulnerable, and we will *all* die—it is imperative that this fundamental virtue be maintained. And that requires, we might say, a medical-moral ecology that upholds the virtue and makes its continued existence possible. Such an ecology requires that the norm against intentionally harming or killing be maintained in the medical profession with all the strictness suggested by the Way of Medicine. That norm is the touchstone of medicine.

CHAPTER TEN

Conscientious Medicine

Doctors often refuse patients' requests—a fact about the practice of medicine so familiar that it is easy to overlook—even when patients request interventions that are legal and permitted by the medical profession.

Doctors' refusals are neither new nor infrequent, and only a small minority occasion any controversy. Surgeons refuse to operate when they believe a surgery is unlikely to succeed. Physicians refuse medications when they believe the medications are unlikely to be helpful. Clinicians refuse requested interventions because of concerns about safety or efficacy, and they refuse because of less tangible concerns that are no less real. Some pediatricians refuse to supplement the growth hormones of boys who are short because of concerns about crossing a line between treatment and enhancement. Some primary care physicians at times refuse costly workups for what they believe are psychosomatic syndromes out of concern for their colleagues' time and other medical resources. Obstetrician-gynecologists who will abort fetuses with lethal congenital anomalies may refuse to abort those with Down syndrome or cleft palates out of concern about societal attitudes toward those with disabilities or those who are female out of concern about sexism. Physicians refuse patients' requests even when such requests are informed, even when patients meet some published criteria for the intervention in question, and even when physicians are aware that some or even most of their colleagues would disagree with their refusals.

In recent years, however, controversy has erupted over the issue of physicians' refusing to provide or facilitate patients' access to certain morally contested interventions, such as abortions, physician-assisted suicides, or surgical modifications of secondary sex characteristics (gender transition services). When physicians refuse such interventions, many now argue, they are letting their personal values interfere with their professional obligations.[1] A recent essay in the *New England Journal of Medicine* by Ronit Stahl and Ezekiel Emanuel illustrates the point: Stahl and Emanuel assert that patients have a right to choose the healthcare services they need for their own *well-being*, and physicians have a corollary obligation to accommodate the patients' choices, either by providing the requested interventions directly or by referring the patients to doctors who will.[2]

Such claims are starting to gain the force of policy in some jurisdictions. Historically, the medical profession has given wide latitude to physicians' discretion in areas of disagreement. Professional codes have consistently stated that physicians are not obligated to satisfy patients' requests for interventions that the physicians believe are not in the interest of the patients' health. In 2015, however, Ontario's College of Physicians and Surgeons issued a rule requiring physicians to "take positive steps" to make "effective referrals" for all legal interventions that a patient might request, including euthanasia. The college's working group concluded that there is "no qualitative difference" between euthanasia and other "health care services."[3] In 2016, the Illinois General Assembly revised a decades-old law that previously had prevented employers from discriminating against healthcare workers who refused to engage in practices to which they had principled objections. The new version requires employees to at least make referrals.[4] In 2017 Sweden's Labor Court ruled that clinics can lawfully refuse work to nurse midwives who refuse to perform abortions.[5] If physicians have personal objections to some interventions, the reasoning goes, they must avoid areas of medicine in which those interventions are likely to be requested.

Something is right about all of this. After all, as Stahl and Emanuel put it, physicians are not conscripts. No one is compelled to become a physician, and in becoming a physician, one willingly takes on responsibilities that go with the role. Surely the profession and the public can hold physicians to fulfill their professional responsibilities or, as Stahl and Emanuel put it, their "role morality."[6] We would not countenance teachers who refuse to grade their students' work or attorneys who refuse to represent their clients before the justice system. Why would we allow physicians to refuse what patients request?

Yet the boundaries of what we accept and what we reject where professional refusals are concerned clearly center on answers to the following questions: what is the profession for, and what are the obligations that come with one's profession? Teachers are allowed and even expected to refuse requests of students if those requests are irrelevant or run contrary to the purposes of teaching. The same is true for lawyers and their clients.

The same is also true for medicine, yet medicine is, as we have argued throughout this book, in the grip of a conflict between two radically different ways of answering these questions, and debates about conscientious refusals indicate that the profession of medicine cannot continue indefinitely with these two contradictory construals of its purpose. The issue of conscientious refusals brings the rivalry and tension between the PSM and the Way of Medicine to a head. Physicians face a choice, and the stakes are high. Insofar as their profession embraces the PSM, physicians' consciences threaten their patients' well-being and must be suppressed. Unfortunately, by suppressing conscientious practice, the PSM reduces medicine to a demoralized job and augurs the end of medicine as a profession. Therefore, we encourage physicians to reject the PSM and recover the profession's orientation to their patients' health as a genuine good. This commitment to their patients' health gives physicians a reasonable standard for discerning which requests should be accommodated and which refused.

The Provider of Services Model and Physicians' Refusal

Abe Anderson's physician refuses to prescribe antibiotics.

Cindy Parker's physician refuses to refer her for an abortion.

In the PSM, informed consent gives way to informed choice: patients choose, physicians provide. A physician may refuse to perform interventions that are technically infeasible, illegal, or unavailable and may refuse interventions that are futile with respect to the reason for which the patient seeks the intervention. But if these threshold conditions are met, the patients' choices are to be accommodated. Principles can be brought to bear, of course, and utilities can be measured in an effort to maximize them. The physician can also advert to "accepted clinical and professional norms." Only the patient, however, is in a position to balance and specify the relevant principles or to weigh the relevant utilities in order to determine what the patient's well-being requires. Moreover, according to the PSM, the central clinical and professional norm is putting patient well-being first; personal scruples cannot get in the way of a patient's receiving what she genuinely believes she needs.

This idea of patient well-being plays a central role in the PSM. When proponents of the PSM criticize conscientious refusals, they consistently refer to the patient's well-being rather than to the patient's health. "Health care *providers*," write Stahl and Emanuel, "have a primary interest: to promote the well-being of patients."[7] And again: according to the American Congress of Obstetrics and Gynecology (ACOG), "Providers" have a "fundamental duty to enable patients to make decisions for themselves."[8] Under the PSM, medical professionals are providers whose goal is to do what is conducive to patients' well-being. This defines what Stahl and Emanuel call the physician's "role morality." Adhering to that morality "means offering and providing accepted medical interventions in accordance with patients' reasoned decisions."[9]

Given all of this, we might expect proponents of the PSM to condemn both of the above refusals. Curiously, that is not what happens. True, Mr. Anderson and Ms. Parker both request interventions that are feasible, legal, and available, and neither intervention is futile with respect to the patient's goals. Moreover, Abe and Cindy both believe their well-being requires the interventions they request. Abe understands why the physician does not recommend antibiotics, but he wants the prescription in order to satisfy his wife and to reduce the (albeit small) risk of his missing more days of work. Cindy understands why many find abortion morally problematic, but she wants the abortion in order to preserve the future that she believes she will lose if she carries the pregnancy to term. Despite these similarities, only the physician's refusal of Cindy's request typically raises the ire of those who criticize conscientious refusals.

How can this be? On the Way of Medicine, each refusal may be justified insofar as it is grounded in a judgment that what is requested does not serve, or indeed is contrary to, the end of patient health. How, though, can the PSM distinguish between the two cases? It does so by introducing and leaning heavily on a new distinction: between refusals based on professional reasons and refusals based on personal reasons. According to the PSM, the physician who refuses Abe's request for antibiotics is justified because the physician refuses for *medical* or *professional* reasons and thereby upholds the physician's "role morality." In contrast, the physician who refuses Cindy's request is condemned for allowing *personal* and *private* concerns to intrude on what should be a strictly professional consideration.

It is difficult to overstate the importance to the PSM of the distinction between the personal and the professional, whether posed as personal moral values versus professional ethical obligations, personal conscience versus professional conscience,[10] personal integrity versus professional integrity,[11] or simply personal reasons versus medical reasons. Physicians may believe what they will "in their private lives," write Stahl and Emanuel, "but in their role as health care professionals, they must provide the appropriate interventions as specified by the medical profession."[12]

It perhaps goes without saying that judgments of conscience are, for the PSM, the apotheosis of the personal. To refuse on the basis of conscience is to allow personal biases to interfere with professional obligations, particularly with the obligation to respect patients' *autonomy*. It may be difficult, the reasoning goes, but sometimes clinicians have professional obligations to do what their personal consciences object to doing.

Yet even advocates of the PSM concede that clinicians may refuse patients' requests when they have strong medical reasons to do so, as presumably Mr. Anderson's physician did, judging that antibiotics are not medically indicated for a viral infection. How does one know whether one's reasons are sufficiently medical? The PSM fails to provide any nonarbitrary standard to guide such judgments (a problem to which we return below), but proponents of the PSM are clear that medical reasons simply cannot include traditional norms such as the injunction to never intentionally damage or destroy the patient's health. They are equally clear that physicians who allow personal concerns to influence their professional practices thereby abuse their power and threaten harm to their patients—not harm to the patients' health per se, but harm to "well-being as the patient perceives it."[13]

Here we see the final conceptual novelty of the PSM: its standard for harm emerges from its standard for benefit—patient well-being. In the end, if the patient desires something in accordance with her conception of her own well-being, the PSM calls on the physician to provide what the patient requests or at least refer her to someone who will. To do otherwise is to fail to obey the principle of nonmaleficence.

This position comes with deep political and professional implications. From the standpoint of social authorities, including the state and professional licensing organizations, the PSM implies that a physician is obligated via an implicit social contract to provide health-care services according to the patient's informed choices. Dan Brock, in arguing that physicians are at least obligated to refer patients for any legal intervention, takes for granted that the medical profession is obligated by social contract to make available all legal interventions.[14] Therefore, authorities must scrutinize physicians' refusals carefully; the burden of proof is on physicians to justify their refusals and to show that they are not based on personal values.

ACOG proposes further scrutiny to make sure that physicians' refusals are not based on prejudice and that they are based on sound science.[15] Physicians may not, for example, refuse to prescribe contraceptives based on concern about preventing implantation of an embryo, because studies suggest that the incidence of such effects is low (there is no need to consider whether the incidence is low enough to make the moral difference, as long as there is "scientific support" for treating the incidence as trivial). Some proponents of the PSM ask policymakers to mandate such scrutiny, to demand alternative service from those who refuse patients' requests,[16] and to threaten sanctions that would make conscientious refusals costly.[17]

But such demands appear to be merely stopgap measures in anticipation of the desired end state: the elimination of conscientious refusals from the professional lives of physicians. As Julian Savulescu put it more than a decade ago in an essay that seems increasingly prophetic, "If people are not prepared to offer legally permitted, efficient, and beneficial care to a patient because it conflicts with their values, they should not be doctors."[18]

The Way of Medicine and Physician Refusal

The Way of Medicine casts physicians' refusals in a very different light, asking first whether a refusal is consistent with, or contradicts, the physicians' commitment to the patients' health. Rather than a prima facie obligation to provide whatever a patient seeks, the physician instead has an obligation to pursue what the patient's health requires (understanding that there may be several possible avenues of pursuit) and to refuse to act in ways that are contrary to the patient's health. Such refusals, rather than abusing power, properly exercise the physician's authority.

Note how differently the Way of Medicine treats the categories of *personal* and *professional*. Because the PSM eschews any objective end for medicine, the professional obligations of the physician must come from outside the practice of medicine. Those obligations cannot be generated and justified by commitments to an objective good that provides the purpose for the profession. Hence the importance of what is legal, what is technically possible, and what is desired by the patient, none of which is intrinsically related to an essential purpose of medicine. Thus also, professional obligations are potentially at odds with the physician's personal commitments, which must be left behind or overcome when they conflict with the "professional."

By contrast, the Way of Medicine calls on the physician, as a member of the profession, to personally deepen and specify a commitment that the physician already has made: attending to those who are sick so as to preserve and restore their health—to raise that commitment to the level appropriate to a vocation-defining profession. For practitioners of medicine, then, the central obligation in each of the above cases is clear: to act reasonably to preserve and restore the patient's health, and to refuse to act otherwise.

As we see from a slightly more philosophical perspective in the next section, physicians can succeed in this task only if they practice according to conscience. A physician's conscience is clinical judgment in action. It is the capacity used when judging whether an inclination to refuse Abe's or Cindy's request is based on good reason, unreasonable desire, or unjustified prejudice. Practicing conscientiously may be difficult, but it can never be reasonable for a clinician to do otherwise.

The Way of Medicine also has implications for those with professional and political authority. It teaches them that if physicians are to attend to those who are sick using reasonable means to preserve and restore their health, they need professional space in which to exercise judgment and to practice conscientiously. Although the state has grounds to hold physicians accountable to general norms of justice and the licensing and accrediting authorities have grounds to hold physicians accountable to meet their professional obligations, neither the state nor any other authority has grounds to compel physicians to contradict their professional responsibilities.

Thus, neither the state nor the profession should be in the business of coercing physicians into meeting unscrutinized patient demands, any more than they should coerce patients to accept this rather than that physician proposal. Patients must be protected from the unscrupulous and the incompetent, which a profession's best efforts will never entirely succeed in weeding out, and a profession must ensure that all its professionals carry out the constitutive commitments of the profession to seek healing for those who are sick. But professional responsibility encompasses the obligation, and hence the right, to make conscientious judgments about what is required in light of one's guiding professional and vocational commitments. This is no less true for physicians than for other professionals.

VIRTUES OF THE WAY OF MEDICINE

One's approach to conscientious refusals turns on how one defines the substance of physicians' professional commitments and obligations, and we have argued throughout the book that the Way of Medicine specifies those commitments and obligations more reasonably. The Way of Medicine has additional virtues that the PSM lacks.

A Better Understanding of Conscience

What makes a refusal *conscientious*? A judgment of conscience is, in the paradigm case, a person's final determination of what is permitted, not permitted, or obligatory in a particular circumstance. What faculty is responsible for these judgments? The traditional view is that of Aquinas: it is *practical reason*, which knows the first principles of the moral law, and *practical reason*, which applies those principles to situations and circumstances so as to lead to particular moral judgments about how one ought to act. Thus, the faculty that is responsible for judgments of conscience, as well as the more general normative judgments presupposed by conscience, is human reason, which is why we have spoken throughout this book of the requirements of practical reason.[19]

Three points are worth noting here. First, conscience judges a person's *own* actions or motives, not those of others. Second, conscience is not a set of considerations that a person might weigh in making a moral judgment; rather, conscience is exercised in the *judgment* about how one should act in light of all such considerations. Third, as an act of human reason, conscience is necessarily limited and fallible; no person sees with absolute clarity, and no person judges his or her own actions with perfect accuracy.

In light of these three points, we can see that although conscientiousness—following one's judgments of conscience—is necessary for ethical action, it is not sufficient. A malformed or misinformed conscience will err. For example, a conscientious physician may fail in his duties to relieve a patient's debilitating pain because he has not been trained to pay close attention to or seek to relieve pain. Alternatively, he may fail because he mistakenly interprets the patients' behavior as drug-seeking and malingering. So every physician is obligated to seek to inform his or her conscience with the best available information, including true moral principles. Every physician must consider arguments made by patients or colleagues that call the physician's initial judgment into question, and physicians must be willing to change their judgment when they can see that it was mistaken.

Nevertheless, in the end physicians must act, and however fallible, physicians can act ethically only if they act according to their consciences. Errors with respect to conscience obscure this fact. According to ACOG, "An appeal to conscience would express a sentiment such as 'If I were to do "*x*," I could not live with myself / I would hate myself / I wouldn't be able to sleep at night.'"[20] In fact, rarely are conscientious practices so emotionally momentous. Rather, to practice conscientiously is simply to act according to one's best judgment about how one ought to act from situation to situation, patient to patient.

Others allege that appeals to conscience are disingenuous and hide unspoken prejudices.[21] It goes without saying that physicians who act disingenuously are not acting conscientiously. To act conscientiously is to act according to what one understands to be the demands of reason. Even where agreement exists about the purposes of medicine, physicians still must consider innumerable different factors in order to discern how best to seek the health of a particular patient in a particular context. This task is almost always attended by ambiguity and uncertainty, requiring what Aristotle called *phronesis* or practical wisdom, the manifestation of which in the practice of medicine has been called good clinical judgment.[22] If physicians are to exercise clinical judgment in seeking their patients' health, they will necessarily refuse some patient requests.

These points illustrate another virtue of the Way of Medicine: its understanding of conscience is much more adequate than that of the PSM. The PSM asks us to treat conscience not as a faculty of reason but as a set of arbitrary and idiosyncratic personal values. Stahl and Emanuel equate conscience with appeal to "personal religious or moral beliefs."[23] With conscience so construed, the physician who acts conscientiously is focused on himself and his own needs rather than on the good and what is required of him. ACOG similarly associates conscientiousness with a need to be able to sleep at night and a defense against moral disintegration. These personal needs, however important, are in tension with one's professional commitments: "By virtue of entering the profession of medicine, physicians accept a set of moral values—and duties—that are central to medical practice. Thus, with professional privileges come *professional responsibilities* to patients, which must precede a provider's *personal interests*."[24] Stahl and Emanuel similarly aver that, "physicians' personal commitments cannot outweigh the interests of patients," and they contend that to follow conscience in refusing a patient's request "violates the central tenet of professional role morality in the field of medicine: the patient comes first."[25]

These misconstruals of what the conscience is lead critics to make unsupportable and contradictory claims. Critics claim that a clinician who refuses a patient's request thereby allows the clinician's conscience to trump the patient's conscience, when in fact no conscience can trump another conscience, since conscience judges only one's own actions. Critics claim that physicians should distinguish "personal conscience" from "professional conscience," or that physicians should balance one or both against other considerations in deciding what to do in a given case.[26] Some critics also suggest that a physician occasionally has an obligation to act against conscience.

Such claims can make sense only if the conscience is a set of values. Then one could have a professional conscience, a personal conscience, and perhaps others as well. One could weigh up the conscience against other considerations, or one conscience against another. One might even have reason to act against conscience. But none of these construals makes sense in light of what the conscience is: the faculty of reason that renders the final judgment as regards what one ought to do, all things considered. So understood, an individual has but one conscience and integrity requires that her conscience cannot be split into components. She cannot take up her judgment of conscience as one consideration among others. While a physician might well have reason to reconsider an initial judgment in light of new information, it can never be right to act against conscience, for in doing so one is acting contrary to one's final judgment about how one ought to act. That is a paradigm case of acting unreasonably.

A Better Understanding of "Professional Responsibility"

The Way of Medicine not only has a more adequate construal of conscience and its place in the practice of medicine than the PSM; it also possesses a nonarbitrary standard for distinguishing refusals that align with the physician's vocation from those that contradict that vocation. Unless we are to say that physicians may never refuse anything patients request, physicians must have some criteria by which to distinguish between justified and unjustified refusals.

The PSM turns, for such criterion, to the putative distinction between the personal and the professional. As we show here, the problem with this putative distinction is that the term *"personal"* has no meaning in these debates except "not professional," and *"not professional"* has no meaning unless one can specify the content of the physician's profession. As Abe's case demonstrates, without an objective standard for the medical profession, saying that a concern is merely personal is not possible. Anything that relates to the patient's well-being can be considered a professional concern.

In the end, the category of "personal" distracts from and cloaks the fact that the PSM cannot say what the physician's profession requires beyond accommodating patients' considered, informed requests for legal and technically feasible interventions. Without any objective standard to look to, proponents of the PSM draw idiosyncratic and arbitrary lines between the personal and the professional. For example, ACOG contends that physicians must refuse policies that require them to report undocumented patients to immigration authorities, because such policies conflict with other professional norms, including the "primary principle of nonmaleficence."[27] In the same piece, however, ACOG takes it for granted that physicians must refer patients for abortion, ignoring altogether arguments that abortion violates the same principle of nonmaleficence. Stahl and Emanuel claim that physicians might justifiably refuse assisted suicide—a practice Emanuel has publicly opposed for decades—because the practice is "currently controversial and subject to debate about whether [it is] medically appropriate."[28] However, they cannot bring themselves to imagine that abortion and gender transition surgery are similarly controversial and subject to similar debate. "Professional" responsibilities thus emerge as sufficiently malleable to rule out what a writer dislikes and to require what the writer affirms.

In seeking to say more about the "professional," proponents of the PSM often look to public and professional opinion in arbitrary and self-contradictory ways or appeal to straw men to critique moral judgments in medicine. On the one hand, they will refer to a "standard of care" and a "consensus" as establishing the scope of what physicians must do. But in the next breath they refer to the absence of consensus as the reason physicians cannot justifiably refuse some intervention (because many people disagree with the physician's "personal" opinion). In a particularly curious turn, Stahl and Emanuel claim that "health care professionals voluntarily choose their roles and thus become obligated to provide, perform, and refer patients for interventions according to the standards of the profession." Yet they then lament that the organizations that most authoritatively establish the standards of the profession "all tend to accept rather than question conscientious objection in health care."[29] ACOG as well as Stahl and Emanuel acknowledges deep societal disagreement about whether abortion is permissible, yet both claim that abortion is standard medical practice. "Although abortion is politically and culturally contested," Stahl and Emanuel write, "it is not medically controversial."[30] So again, in the absence of clarity about the professional commitments of medicine, proponents sometimes rely on and sometimes disavow claims of consensus and controversy, adopting a whatever-works strategy in an attempt to force their desired shape of conformity onto the profession.

The Way of Medicine, by contrast, distinguishes not between the professional and the personal but between that which fulfills the physician's profession and that which departs from or contradicts that profession. In an important sense, this merely distinguishes the reasonable from the unreasonable, with attention to the particular vocation of practitioners of medicine.

Critics worry that physicians' refusals hide invidious discrimination under the guise of conscience. Stahl and Emanuel say that to refuse to participate in "gender reassignment surgery, or the use of contraception . . . is to allow personal moral judgment to masquerade as medical practice."[31] ACOG contends, "Finally, conscientious refusals should be evaluated on the basis of their potential for discrimination."[32] But the Way of Medicine can coherently condemn refusals that involve invidious discrimination without abandoning either the notion of conscience or the physicians' commitment to the patient's health.

The physician who refuses to care for patients with HIV because of antipathy toward homosexuals or for patients of another race because of racial prejudice or for criminals because of revulsion at their crimes violates the constitutive professional obligation to seek the health of patients precisely because they are sick, without regard to their other characteristics. After all, the good of health is good for all persons. The professional obligation to seek the health of patients is to be contrasted not with conscience or with personal obligations but instead with failures of reason. The solution to such failures is, in fact, sound exercise of conscience.

A Greater Respect for Pluralism

In contrast with the PSM, the Way of Medicine presents a workable, peaceable approach to living with disagreement—with the pluralism that defines our current age. Stahl and Emanuel, speaking for the PSM, write, "Health care professionals who are unwilling to accept these limits [to conscientious refusals] have two choices: select an area of medicine, such as radiology, that will not put them in situations that conflict with their personal morality or, if there is no such area, leave the profession."[33]

If the profession followed this logic to its conclusion, it would have to drum out those who have the audacity to refuse interventions because they are not required by or conducive to the patients' health. This is a recipe for a homogenous and authoritarian healthcare profession, one held together by the forcible imposition of external norms: the norms of the legally permitted, the technologically feasible, and what patients desire. Physicians unwilling to work within these constraints would have to go.

Perhaps paradoxically, the Way of Medicine has much more flexibility. Let us grant the "fact of reasonable pluralism."[34] There is, we concede, no way to recover (or forge anew) full agreement on the part of all physicians regarding the moral obligations of medical practitioners. Nevertheless, if we imagine a profession structured even minimally on a commitment to patients' health, the profession should allow conscientious refusals where reasoned dispute exists about whether an intervention is consistent with that goal.

In such circumstances, patients may face clinicians who make clear, in so many words, that they do not believe what the patient seeks is what the clinician should be doing. Patients in some areas, particularly rural areas, may struggle to find clinicians who will provide interventions that are available elsewhere. The profession will sustain in its ranks an ongoing contention about what good medicine requires. The presence of differences will push people to consider why they are making the choices they make rather than taking practices for granted. Physicians will represent the diversity of moral communities found in a society, and the range of choices among philosophies of care will reflect the ongoing moral disagreements among those communities. When people like Stahl and Emanuel insist that physicians put their professional obligations first, we will insist that they make an argument to show how physicians' commitment to their patients' health, objectively construed, requires them to participate in the interventions in question.

We are optimistic that such a profession would come to recognize again that certain practices are simply incompatible with physicians' commitment to patients' health. Abortion, euthanasia, and sex reassignment surgeries, for example, would be seen as simply not the business of physicians, though treatment of pregnant mothers and their infant children, the dying, and those suffering from gender dysphoria would be. There would still be considerable room for disagreement, given the complexity of health and the vagueness and indeterminacy around its boundaries—and that is to say nothing of the scope for disagreement over how best to address the health of a particular patient, given the inevitable limitations of medical knowledge and technology.

The Way of Medicine recognizes that a profession must have something that its practitioners *profess* in common; that something, for medicine, is the patient's health. The PSM gives, by contrast, a merely formal shared end: the satisfaction of patients' desires within what the law and medical science allow, a goal that will frequently lead physicians to pursue contradictory ends—for example, the life of this fetus, the death of that one. But within the pursuit of health, the Way of Medicine sees room for professional comity and amity: comity when the conscientious judgments of other physicians are respected and amity when the profession is willing to tolerate diverse moral and religious views if those are not essentially unjust. That is a far cry from the PSM's increasingly aggressive intolerance of disagreement.

THE FUTURE OF MEDICINE

Elevating the PSM over the Way of Medicine will lead to three logical if unintended consequences. First, any policy that constrains the scope of conscientious refusals will thereby erode the possibility of conscientious practice. It seems obvious that patients want their physicians to be conscientious insofar as possible. Who wants a physician who is in the habit of doing what he knows he should not do? Fortunately, individuals from virtually all moral traditions and communities can conscientiously commit themselves to caring for the sick. That is one reason the profession of medicine has been able to maintain prestige and a measure of unity in a society comprising many different moral communities. Yet efforts to reduce the scope of conscientious refusals will gradually squeeze out or block from entry all but those who are willing to make available to patients the full range of legal technological interventions and to set aside their judgments about which interventions are congruent with patients' health.

Consider obstetrics and gynecology. If the PSM prevails, the obstetrics and gynecology practice of the future will be hospitable only to those willing to engage in elective abortion, sterilization, contraception, IVF, prenatal genetic diagnosis, surrogate pregnancy, artificial insemination, cosmetic genital surgery, gender transition surgery, and whatever comes next. Only a minority of American physicians can cooperate conscientiously in all of these legal, feasible, and yet morally controversial practices. Paradoxically, patients' choices will be reduced insofar as they will not be able to seek out trained clinicians who share their judgment that such practices contradict the purposes of medicine. So the process will go. Every time the scope of conscientious refusal is narrowed, the pool of people who can be conscientious physicians is reduced.

The second consequence is that by requiring physicians to do what patients request, policies that constrain the scope of physician refusals will put physicians and patients at odds with one another. The PSM already treats the physician's judgment as a threat to the patient. If physicians cannot refuse patient requests, they will wonder when their patients might, with the backing of legal sanction, ask them to act against their own understanding and do that which they believe is unethical. By making physicians obey patients, we will make patients a moral threat to their physicians.

The third consequence of reducing the scope of conscientious refusals is that patients will lose the basis for trusting that their physicians are committed to their good. Under the old model of paternalism, patients could trust that physicians had committed themselves to their patients' best interests, albeit in a limited way—only insofar as those interests included restoring and preserving health. The patients' rights movement and the doctrine of informed consent rightly qualified and delimited physicians' commitment to pursue health. Out of respect for the persons they serve, physicians are to act only with the permission of their patients. Because health is neither the only nor the highest good, patients are authorized to situate that good in relation to other concerns such as not being overburdened by medical technology.

The PSM differs fundamentally: in it, patients not only qualify how their health will be pursued but also decide what outcomes and states of affairs their physicians will seek. Patients gain technicians committed to cooperation and lose healers committed to their good. They gain control over physicians but thereby divest physicians of responsibility. As a result, patients will "often navigate treacherous medical terrain without adequate medical guidance."[35] Physicians can wash their hands of patients' decisions, as long as they give their patients accurate information and provide technically proficient "healthcare services."

By asking physicians to set aside their consciences and detach from their historical commitment to their patients' health, the PSM contributes to a crisis of medical morale, because the PSM quite literally demoralizes medicine. If medicine merely provides desired services to maximize patients' vision of well-being, medicine's pretense to moral seriousness will be a charade and its attempts at professionalism a façade. Is it surprising that today's physicians, conditioned to think of themselves largely as mere functionaries, suffer high rates of burnout?[36]

There is a better way. That way involves conscientiousness and candor on the part of physicians. Where there is ambiguity or a dispute arises about whether a particular practice belongs in medicine, physicians and patients can do their best to negotiate an accommodation that does not require either to do what they believe is unethical. Rather than feign moral neutrality, physicians will tell their patients frankly what their options are, which ones the physician is willing to offer, and why the physician recommends one over another. The scope of permissible accommodations will have to be set through the political process, but we echo the conclusion reached by the President's Commission way back in 1982: "Considerable flexibility should be accorded to patients and professionals to define the terms of their own relationships."[37]

In conclusion, unless and until consensus is forged regarding the ends of medicine, refusals of controversial practices cannot be shown to violate physicians' professional obligations. In the meantime, the practice of medicine should be open to anyone who is willing to unreservedly commit him- or herself to caring for the sick so as to preserve and restore their health.

WORKING FOR HEALTH, CONTENDING FOR MEDICINE

We close by calling for healthcare professionals to strive conscientiously for their patients' health and in so doing to contend conscientiously for good medicine. In some contexts, practicing the Way of Medicine will require courage, even great courage. Trailblazers must sometimes walk alone. As Martin Luther King Jr. said, "There comes a time when one must take a position that is neither safe, nor politic, nor popular, but he must take it because conscience tells him it is right."[38]

We do not suggest that everyone who finds the Way of Medicine compelling should immediately set out to persuade every proponent of the PSM that they are in error. Some are called to that task, but certainly not all are. Nor do we recommend that physicians contend for their "rights"; we are not advocating the antagonism of "rights talk" or pitting physicians' rights against those of patients.

Rather, our suggestion is to practice medicine according to reason and to be prepared to give an account of why you do what you do. Be committed to the central good of medicine: patient health. Do nothing contrary to that good, and align your practice to be in harmony with that good. Cultivate the virtues of good medicine. Be a physician and a healer, not merely a technician or a provider.

In short, be a *good* physician, practicing good medicine. Doing so will function to the good of your patients and to your good as a doctor. It may also persuade your colleagues and patients. As Leon Kass has noted, the most basic truths often are better demonstrated in practice than in argument.[39] By pursuing their patients' health in time-tested ways that respect the moral law, clinicians show others a better way of caring for their patients — a way that has an integrity and even a beauty that may win over those who at present are captive to the PSM.

Clinicians are not alone in this endeavor. This has been a book of medical ethics, and medical ethicists and policymakers also must discern the shape of the true practice of medicine and recognize its counterfeits. In providing resources for that task, we hope to have made a modest contribution to the renewal of medicine — a moral project that is ever worthy and ever incomplete.

PREFACE

1. David L. Sackett, William M. C. Rosenberg, J. A. Muir Gray, R. Brian Haynes, and W. Scott Richardson, "Evidence-Based Medicine: What It Is and What It Isn't," *British Medical Journal* 312, no. 7023 (1996): 71–72.

INTRODUCTION

1. It is important for us to clarify our use of "well-being" here. Our own moral theory has a substantive account of human flourishing at its foundations, and such flourishing could equally be designated as a form of well-being. However, throughout this book, when we use the expression in *italics*—*well-being*—we mean to designate the thin, preference- and desire-satisfaction model that many medical ethicists presently use. We typically italicize the first use of the expression in a chapter, and then rely on context to make it clear which sense of "well-being" we mean.

2. As we discuss further in chapter 1, Beauchamp and Childress's enormously influential framework focuses on four principles: beneficence, nonmaleficence, justice, and autonomy. See Tom L. Beauchamp and James F. Childress, *Principles of Biomedical Ethics*, 7th ed. (New York: Oxford University Press, 2013), 13–14.

3. See Ronit Y. Stahl and Ezekiel J. Emanuel, "Physicians, Not Conscripts—Conscientious Objection in Health Care," *New England Journal of Medicine* 376, no. 14 (2017): 1380–85.

4. H. Tristram Engelhardt, *The Foundations of Bioethics*, 2nd ed. (New York: Oxford University Press, 1996), 7.

5. A 2016 *U.S. News & World Report* article showed that "nearly half of U.S. physicians—49 percent—meet the definition for overall burnout." In

addition, physicians' "satisfaction with work-life balance is far lower than that of others: 36 percent versus 61 percent." See Steve Sternberg, "Diagnosis: Burnout," *U.S. News & World Report*, September 8, 2016. See also Tait D. Shanafelt, Omar Hasan, Lotte N. Dyrbye, Christine Sinsky, Daniel Satele, Jeff Sloan, and Colin P. West, "Changes in Burnout and Satisfaction with Work-Life Balance in Physicians and the General US Working Population between 2011 and 2014," *Mayo Clinic Proceedings* 90, no. 12 (2015): 1600–1613.

6. Michael J. Balboni and Tracy A. Balboni, *Hostility to Hospitality: Spirituality and Professional Socialization within Medicine* (New York: Oxford University Press, 2019).

7. As will become clear, we see two interrelated disagreements about medicine: one over whether health should be the primary and largely exclusive purpose of medicine and one over what health is.

8. Edelstein's translation renders the Greek well: "I will neither give a deadly drug to anybody if asked for it, nor will I make a suggestion to this effect. Similarly I will not give to a woman an abortive remedy" (οὐ δώσω δὲ οὐδὲ φάρμακον οὐδενὶ αἰτηθεὶς θανάσιμον οὐδὲ ὑφηγήσομαι ξυμβουλίην τοιήδε· ὁμοίως δὲ οὐδὲ γυναικὶ πεσσὸν φθόριον δώσω). Ludwig Edelstein, *The Hippocratic Oath: Text, Translation, and Interpretation* (Baltimore, MD: Johns Hopkins University Press, 1943), 2–3.

9. For discussion of this claim in relation to the oath itself, see T. A. Cavanaugh, *Hippocrates' Oath and Asclepius' Snake* (New York: Oxford University Press, 2018).

10. C. S. Lewis, *The Abolition of Man, or, Reflections on Education with Special Reference to the Teaching of English in the Upper Forms of Schools* (San Francisco: HarperSanFrancisco, 2001), 43.

11. Gerald P. McKenney, *To Relieve the Human Condition: Bioethics, Technology, and the Body* (Albany, NY: State University of New York [SUNY] Press, 1997), 16. McKenney himself engages dialectically with a number of previous critics, such as Hans Jonas Leon Kass and Stanley Hauerwas, from whom we have also learned much.

12. Jeffrey P. Bishop, *The Anticipatory Corpse: Medicine, Power, and the Care of the Dying* (Notre Dame, IN: University of Notre Dame Press, 2011).

13. Ibid., 9.

14. "Social imaginary" is a term that Charles Taylor explores in depth in his *Modern Social Imaginaries* (Durham, NC: Duke University Press, 2004), 23.

15. Edmund D. Pellegrino, "The Internal Morality of Clinical Medicine: A Paradigm for the Ethics of the Helping and Healing Professions," *Journal of Medicine and Philosophy* 26, no. 6 (2001): 559–79.

16. McKenney, *To Relieve the Human Condition: Bioethics*, 16.

17. See Edmund D. Pellegrino, *The Philosophy of Medicine Reborn: A Pellegrino Reader*, ed. H. Tristram Engelhardt Jr. and Fabrice Jotterand (Notre Dame, IN: University of Notre Dame Press, 2008); Leon R. Kass, "Regarding the End of Medicine and the Pursuit of Health," *Public Interest* 4 (1975): 11–42; Alasdair MacIntyre, *After Virtue: A Study in Moral Theology*, 3rd ed. (Notre Dame, IN: University of Notre Dame Press, 2007), 194. See also John Keown's assessment of John Finnis: "A New Father for the Law and Ethics of Medicine," in Robert P. George and John Keown, *Reason, Morality, and Law: The Philosophy of John Finnis* (Oxford: Oxford University Press, 2014), 290–307.

18. See MacIntyre, *After Virtue*, 222.

CHAPTER ONE   The Way of Medicine

1. Alasdair MacIntyre, *After Virtue: A Study in Moral Theory*, 3rd ed. (Notre Dame, IN: University of Notre Dame Press, 2007), 187.

2. For more on the difference between experiencing one's work as a job versus as a calling, see Robert N. Bellah, William M. Sullivan, Richard Madsen, Ann Swindler, and Steven M. Tipton, *Habits of the Heart: Individualism and Commitment in American Life* (Berkeley: University of California Press, 1985); Amy Wrzesniewski, Clark McCauler, Paul Rozin, and Barry Schwartz, "Jobs, Careers, and Callings: People's Relations to Their Work," *Journal of Research in Personality* 31, no. 1 (1997): 21–33; and Douglas T. Hall and Dawn E. Chandler, "Psychological Success: When the Career Is a Calling," *Journal of Organizational Behavior* 26, no. 2 (2005): 155–76.

3. Aristotle, *Nicomachean Ethics*, trans. David Ross (New York: Oxford University Press, 2009), 1094a10.

4. For an introduction to debates about whether medicine has an intrinsic telos and an internal morality, see the collection of papers on the subject in the *Journal of Medicine and Philosophy* 26, no. 6 (2001).

5. See Jean Bethke Elshtain, "Why Science Cannot Stand Alone," *Theoretical Medicine and Bioethics* 29, no. 3 (2008): 161–69.

6. See Paul A. Lombardo, *Three Generations, No Imbeciles: Eugenics, the Supreme Court, and* Buck v. Bell (Baltimore, MD: Johns Hopkins University Press, 2010).

7. Aristotle, *Nicomachean Ethics*, 1094b25.

8. See, particularly, Leon Kass, "Regarding the End of Medicine and the Pursuit of Health," *Public Interest* 40 (1975): 11–42. See also Luke Gormally,

"The Good of Health and the Ends of Medicine," in Holder Zaborowski, *Natural Moral Law in Contemporary Society* (Washington, DC: Catholic University of America Press, 2010), 264–84. Gormally argues for views of both health and medicine very similar to ours.

9. See Christopher Boorse, "Health as a Theoretical Concept," *Philosophy of Science* 44 (1977): 542–73. Some proponents of an objective account, such as Boorse, further understand health as merely the absence of disease. In contrast, we claim that health is a positive quality and is, in this important sense, prior to disease. Disease is knowable because it causes a diminishment of health, but health is knowable apart from any disease. What's more, health can be diminished even in the absence of disease, as when a person becomes unhealthy as a consequence of inactivity. Therefore, the opposite of health is not disease but ill health—the privation or absence of health.

10. For a discussion of evaluative concepts of health and disease see Jacob Stegenga, *Care and Cure: An Introduction to Philosophy of Medicine* (Chicago: University of Chicago Press, 2018), chaps. 1 and 2.

11. These syndromes include conditions such as chronic fatigue and fibromyalgia. See Jiwon Helen Shin, John D. Yoon, Kenneth A. Rasinski, Harold G. Koenig, Keith G. Meador, and Farr A. Curlin, "A Spiritual Problem? Primary Care Physicians' and Psychiatrists' Interpretations of Medically Unexplained Symptoms," *Journal of General Internal Medicine* 28, no. 3 (2013): 392–98.

12. Because humans are ever incomplete, to be human is to be disabled and dependent in significant measure, even if that dependence and disability are not socially conspicuous.

13. Gerald P. McKenny, *To Relieve the Human Condition: Bioethics, Technology, and the Body* (Albany, NY: State University of New York [SUNY] Press, 1997).

14. Some have interpreted Kass as disregarding mental health. He was at pains to distinguish pursuit of happiness from pursuit of health, but in our view, his account of the well-working of the organism as a whole includes mental health in the way we offer here.

15. Kass, "Regarding the End of Medicine," 14; "Constitution of WHO: Principles," World Health Organization, April 7, 1948, https://www.who .int/about/mission/en/.

16. Wendell Berry, "Health Is Membership," in M. Therese Lysaught, Joseph Kotva, Stephen E. Lammers, and Allen Verhey, ed. *On Moral Medicine* (Grand Rapids, MI: Eerdmans, 2012), 420.

17. "Shalom" translates as "peace," but, much like the term "health," "shalom" can be used analogically to refer to wholeness, completeness, and

blessedness. We find it notable that Jewish tradition requires Jews to live in a community that has a physician, and although rabbis can also be physicians—and often have been—Jewish tradition distinguishes the two roles. See Immanuel Jakovovitz, *Jewish Medical Ethics: A Comparative and Historical Study of the Jewish Religious Attitude to Medicine and Its Practice* (New York: Block Publishing, 1975), 204–13.

18. Or, as Kass puts it, "in accordance with its specific excellences," in "Regarding the End of Medicine," 29.

CHAPTER TWO   The Requirements of Practical Reason

1. Aristotle, *Nicomachean Ethics*, trans. David Ross (New York: Oxford University Press, 2009).

2. We think of life and health as constituting one (complex) good. When health is gone, no life remains. When life is present, some health remains. In this book, wherever we use the term "health," we mean this complex basic good of life and health.

3. A commitment to human goods and human flourishing characterizes much natural law theory, yet different theorists identify different goods as basic or fundamental. Our list of basic goods is largely drawn from Germain Grisez, Joseph Boyle, and John Finnis, "Practical Principles, Moral Truth, and Ultimate Ends," *American Journal of Jurisprudence* 32 (1987): 106–8, which, however, omits marriage. That good is present in Aquinas's list in *Summa Theologiae*, 1–2, q. 94, a.2.

4. For a consequentialist approach to some important questions of medical ethics, see Helga Kuhse and Peter Singer, *Should the Baby Live? The Problem of Handicapped Infants* (Oxford: Oxford University Press, 1985). John Harris is an important defender of a broadly libertarian-consequentialist approach to bioethics. See, e.g., Harris, *The Value of Life* (New York: Routledge, 1995).

5. For further discussion, see Robert P. George and Christopher Tollefsen, *Embryo: A Defense of Human Life* (New York: Doubleday, 2008), chap. 4: "Moral Philosophy and the Early Human Being," 83–111.

6. See Rachel Aviv, "What Does It Mean to Die?" *New Yorker*, February 5, 2018, www.newyorker.com.

7. National Commission for the Protection of Human Subjects of Biomedical and Behavioral Research, "The Belmont Report," Department of Health, Education, and Welfare, April 18, 1979, www.hhs.gov.

8. Beauchamp and Childress's first edition of *Principles of Biomedical Ethics* was published in 1979. The book is now in its seventh edition and has for decades been the most widely used medical ethics textbook in the world.

9. Beauchamp refers to all of these as "alleged competitors" of principlism in "Principlism and Its Alleged Competitors," *Kennedy Institute of Ethics Journal* 5, no. 3 (1995).

10. Beauchamp is quite explicit that there are no absolutes and that the prohibition against killing is just the sort of prohibition an ethics needs to be able to overcome (e.g., through compassionate aid-in-dying). See Beauchamp, "Principlism and Its Alleged Competitors."

11. Alfonso Gomez-Lobo also makes, and extends, a similar criticism of principlism in his (with John Keown), *Bioethics and the Human Goods: An Introduction to Natural Law Bioethics* (Washington, DC: Georgetown University Press, 2015).

12. Immanuel Kant, *Grounding for the Metaphysics of Morals.*, trans. James W. Ellington, 3rd ed. (Indianapolis: Hackett, 1993 [1785]), 36.

13. John Rawls, "The Idea of Public Reason Revisited," *University of Chicago Law Review* 60, no. 3 (1997): 765–807.

14. A 2003 survey of US physicians from all specialties found that 71 percent agreed (32 percent strongly) with the statement "For me, the practice of medicine is a calling." See Farr A. Curlin, Lydia S. Dugdale, John D. Lantos, and Marshall H. Chin, "Do Religious Physicians Disproportionately Care for the Underserved?" *Annals of Family Medicine* 5, no. 4 (2007): 353–60. Among those who indicated that they have no religion, 52 percent agreed (20 percent strongly), and among those who indicated that they never attend religious services, 56 percent agreed (22 percent strongly) (data unpublished). A 2010 survey of U.S. primary care physicians and psychiatrists found that more than 80 percent of both groups agreed (about 40 percent strongly) with the same statement. See John D. Yoon, Jiwon H. Shin, Andy L. Nian, and Farr A. Curlin, "Religion, Sense of Calling, and the Practice of Medicine: Findings from a National Survey of Primary Care Physicians and Psychiatrists," *Southern Medical Journal* 108, no. 3 (2015): 189–95. Again, substantial majorities of the unreligious agreed (more than 65 percent of physicians who report no religious affiliation, indicate that they have no religion, and/or indicate that they never attend religious services) (data unpublished).

15. *Gaudium et spes*, no. 24. See *Vatican Council II: The Basic Sixteen Documents; Constitutions, Decrees, Declarations*, rev. ed., ed. Austin Flannery (Northport, NY: Costello Publishing, 1996), 190.

16. For an accessible introduction to the idea of personal vocation, see Germain Grisez and Russell Shaw, *Personal Vocation: God Calls Everyone* (Huntington, IN: Our Sunday Visitor, 2003).

CHAPTER THREE   The Doctor-Patient Relationship

1. Here we focus on the contributions of Mark Siegler as well as Timothy E. Quill and Howard Brody, but there have been many critiques of making patient autonomy the regulative principle for medical ethics. Prominent contributions to this literature include Carl Schneider, *The Practice of Autonomy: Patients, Doctors, and Medical Decisions* (New York: Oxford University Press, 1998); Ezekiel J. Emanuel and Linda L. Emanuel, "Four Models of the Physician-Patient Relationship," *Journal of the American Medical Association* 267, no. 16 (1992): 2221–26; and David Thomasma, "Beyond Medical Paternalism and Patient Autonomy: A Model of Physician Conscience for the Physician-Patient Relationship," *Annals of Internal Medicine* 98, no. 2 (1983): 243–48.

2. Leon R. Kass, "Regarding the End of Medicine and the Pursuit of Health," *Public Interest* 4 (1975): 11–42.

3. Mark Siegler, "Searching for Moral Certainty in Medicine: A Proposal for a New Model of the Doctor-Patient Encounter," *Bulletin of the New York Academy of Medicine* 57, no. 1 (1981): 56–69.

4. Ibid., 58.

5. President's Commission for the Study of Ethical Problems in Medicine and Biomedical and Behavioral Research, "Making Health Care Decisions: The Ethical and Legal Implications of Informed Consent in the Patient-Practitioner Relationship," October 1982, 35, https://repository.library.georgetown.edu.

6. Some physicians can fail in this way for a long time and still be quite useful to patients with respect to health, particularly subspecialists whose work is more reducible to technique and technological production. One thinks, for example, of the brain surgeon who is exquisitely committed to doing a technically proficient job — even a job that deserves to be called "beautiful," but who could not care less about his patients' flourishing. A patient might reasonably seek out such a surgeon, even over the surgeon who fasts and prays for the healing of the patients he carries in his heart, if the latter surgeon is not as technically gifted.

7. Somewhat paradoxically, while the PSM embraces physicians' engaging in practices that violate traditional boundaries by damaging health, it also opposes physicians engaging in practices such as praying with patients, because these practices, while not injuring health, putatively cross professional boundaries. See Farr A. Curlin and Daniel E. Hall, "Strangers or Friends? A Proposal for a New Spirituality-in-Medicine Ethic," *Journal of General Internal Medicine* 20, no. 4 (2005): 370–74, for a deeper analysis of debates about physicians paying attention to the spiritual concerns of patients.

CHAPTER FOUR   Autonomy and Authority

1. The 1979 Belmont Report and the 1982 "Making Health Care Decisions" report both focused on the importance of informed consent—the former with respect to the research context, the latter with respect to clinical practice. See National Commission for the Protection of Human Subjects of Biomedical and Behavioral Research, "The Belmont Report," Department of Health, Education, and Welfare, April 18, 1979, www.hhs.gov. See also President's Commission for the Study of Ethical Problems in Medicine and Biomedical and Behavioral Research, "Making Health Care Decisions: The Ethical and Legal Implications of Informed Consent in the Patient-Practitioner Relationship," October 1982, 35, https://repository.library.georgetown.edu.

2. Immanuel Kant, *Grounding for the Metaphysics of Morals*, trans. James W. Ellington, 3rd ed. (Indianapolis: Hackett, 1993 [1785]), 30.

3. A different formulation of the categorical imperative was cited in chapter 2; Kant believed them to be equivalent despite their apparent differences.

4. For the term "expressive individualism," see Robert N. Bellah, William M. Sullivan, Richard Madsen, Ann Swindler, and Steven M. Tipton, *Habits of the Heart: Individualism and Commitment in American Life* (Berkeley: University of California Press, 1985), 27.

5. For an accessible philosophical history of this cultural emphasis on authentic self-expression and self-development, see Charles Taylor, *The Ethics of Authenticity* (Cambridge, MA: Harvard University Press, 1991).

6. *Planned Parenthood of Southeastern Pennsylvania v. Casey*, 505 U.S. 833 (SCOTUS, 1992), 861.

7. Stephen Darwall, "Two Kinds of Respect," *Ethics* 88, no. 1 (1977): 36–49.

8. Ms. Maynard was a young woman from California who moved to Oregon to die by physician-assisted suicide. We discuss her case further in chapter 9. See Britanny Maynard, "My Right to Death with Dignity at 29," CNN, November 2, 2014, www.cnn.com.

9. See, for example, Health Occupations—Conversion Therapy for Minors—Prohibition (Youth Mental Health Protection Act), Annotated Code of Maryland, Article—Health Occupations, Section 1–212.1.

10. See Ronit Y. Stahl, and Ezekiel J. Emanuel, "Physicians, Not Conscripts—Conscientious Objection in Health Care," *New England Journal of Medicine* 376, no. 14 (2017): 1380–85.

11. For further discussion of this point, see Robert P. George, *Making Men Moral: Civil Liberties and Public Morality* (Oxford: Oxford University Press, 1995), chap. 6.

12. Of course, patients' medical conditions frequently impair their autonomy, sometimes to the point that they cannot be said to be self-governing. How physicians should respond to and care for such patients is a topic we return to in chapter 8.

13. John Finnis, *Natural Law and Natural Rights* (Oxford: Oxford University Press, 2011), 232.

14. Mark Siegler, "Searching for Moral Certainty in Medicine: A Proposal for a New Model of the Doctor-Patient Encounter," *Bulletin of the New York Academy of Medicine* 57, no. 1 (1981): 56–69.

15. For further discussion of this question, see Joseph Boyle, "Personal Responsibility and Freedom in Health Care: A Natural Law Perspective," in *Persons and Their Bodies: Rights, Responsibilities, Relationships*, ed. Mark Cherry (Dordrecht, Netherlands: Springer, 1999): 111–41.

16. We return to these ideas in our discussion of medical decisions at the end of life in chapters 8 and 9.

17. See Timothy E. Quill and Howard Brody, "Physician Recommendations and Patient Autonomy: Finding a Balance between Physician Power and Patient Choice," *Annals of Internal Medicine* 125, no. 9 (1996): 763–69.

CHAPTER FIVE   The Rule of Double Effect

1. Are there other standards? We think that there are, but that many standards are in one way or another reducible to fairness or vocation. So, for example, one's having promised something bears on what is and is not a proportionate reason for doing that thing; but the importance of promising clearly is related to both fairness and vocation.

2. In some cases, prioritizing is built into a good's nature. Marriage, for example, requires prioritizing marriage above some other goods, and the good of religion, as we argue, requires that religion be put before all other commitments.

3. This way of understanding intention is simpler than that put forth by some philosophers, who, with Thomas Aquinas, identify an "interior object" and an "exterior object" of the human act roughly, where we talk only about "ends" and "means." Nevertheless, we think that our concept largely tracks traditional natural law discussions of intention. Aquinas himself frequently speaks as we do: intention encompasses the end and the means. This simplicity bears fruit, as we discuss below, in our simple formulation of the rule of double effect.

4. Fairness may seem obvious. But vocation? We think so, as it may be that the explorers, recognizing the need for teamwork and trust, have solemnly

promised to one another to "leave no man behind" even if by keeping this promise they will all die. Our point is not that such a commitment is wise but that commitments can specify obligations that reasonably prevent us from doing what we would do if we had not made such commitments.

5. Christopher Tollefsen, "Is a Purely First Person Account of Human Action Defensible?" *Ethical Theory and Moral Practice* 9, no. 4 (2006): 441–60, and Tollefsen, "Double Effect and Two Hard Cases in Medical Ethics," *American Catholic Philosophical Quarterly* 89, no. 3 (2015): 407–20.

6. Sulmasy and Pellegrino describe these four conditions in the following way: "The traditional rule of double effect specifies that an action with 2 possible effects, one good and one bad, is morally permitted if the action: (1) is not in itself immoral, (2) is undertaken only with the intention of achieving the possible good effect, without intending the possible bad effect even though it may be foreseen, (3) does not bring about the possible good effect by means of the possible bad effect, and (4) is undertaken for a proportionately grave reason." Daniel P. Sulmasy and Edmund D. Pellegrino, "The Rule of Double Effect: Clearing Up the Double Talk," *Archives of Internal Medicine* 159, no. 6 (1999): 545–50.

7. See, for example, Timothy E. Quill, Rebecca Dresser, and Dan W. Brock, "The Rule of Double Effect—A Critique of Its Role in End-of-Life Decision Making," *New England Journal of Medicine* 337, no. 24 (1997): 1768–71.

CHAPTER SIX   Sexuality and Reproduction

1. The FDA approved the first oral contraceptive in 1960. For a history of the oral contraceptive, see Bernard Asbell, *The Pill: A Biography of the Drug That Changed the World* (New York: Random House, 1995).

2. Mark Siegler and Dudley Goldblatt, "Clinical Intuition: A Procedure for Balancing the Rights of Patients and the Responsibilities of Physicians," in *The Law—Medicine Relation: A Philosophical Exploration*, ed. S. F. Spicker, J. M. Healey, and H. T. Engelhardt (Dordrecht, Netherlands: Springer, 1981), 25–26.

3. See T. A. Cavanaugh, *Hippocrates' Oath and Asclepius' Snake* (New York: Oxford University Press, 2018), chap. 1.

4. *Planned Parenthood of Southeastern Pennsylvania v. Casey*, 505 U.S. 833 (SCOTUS, 1992), 856.

5. Part of the argument for contraception is that it will reduce the number of abortions by reducing the number of unplanned pregnancies. That seems

intuitive enough, but evidence suggests that abortion rates decline only among users of contraception methods that have very low failure rates and make few demands on users (e.g., intrauterine devices and implantable contraceptives). More common methods, including the oral contraceptive pill, do not seem to reduce abortion rates, and in some cases are associated with higher abortion rates. See William Saletan, "Does Contraception Reduce Abortions?" *Slate*, September 1, 2015, www.slate.com.

6. A prominent website for these practitioners states, "Unlike common suppressive or destructive approaches, NaProTECHNOLOGY works cooperatively with the procreative and gynecologic systems. When these systems function abnormally, NaProTECHNOLOGY *identifies the problems and cooperates* with the menstrual and fertility cycles that correct the condition, maintain the human ecology, and sustain the procreative potential" (emphasis in original). See "NaProTECHNOLOGY," Pope Paul VI Institute for the Study of Human Reproduction, www.naprotechnology.com/.

7. Oliver O'Donovan, Ali Al Chami, and Melanie Davies, "Ovarian Hyperstimulation Syndrome," *Obstetrics, Gynaecology, and Reproductive Medicine* 25, no. 2 (2015): 43–48.

8. See Christopher Tollefsen, "In Vitro Fertilization Should Not Be an Option for a Woman," in *Contemporary Debates in Bioethics*, ed. Arthur L. Caplan and Robert Arp (Chichester, UK: John Wiley & Sons, 2014), 451–59.

9. What Jules and patients like him hope for must be distinguished, of course, from medical attempts to repair damaged secondary sex characteristics and sexual capacities, including attempts to resolve sex ambiguity. More on that below.

10. This distinction has applications outside the natural order also. For example, Thomas Aquinas gives us an account of law as an ordinance of reason, given by one with authority, for the common good, and promulgated. This is the paradigm case, law in good working order. But it is easy to find examples of law that do not share all these features of the paradigm. To pick an obvious example, Jim Crow laws that enforced segregation in the American South did not display these features and as such do not stand as evidence of the diversity of law, properly understood, as much as one among many sordid examples of the distortion of law into something that has the appearance of law but contradicts its purpose. Our capacity to recognize this distinction makes it possible for us to see how unjust laws can, in many circumstances, be justly broken.

11. Kenneth Miller, "Together Forever," *LIFE*, April 1, 1996, 44–54.

12. Congenital vaginal agenesis is a rare condition (experienced by about 1 in 4,000 females) in which a vagina does not form properly before birth.

Reconstructive surgeries can be performed to fashion a vagina. See G. Creatsas and E. Deligeoroglou, "Vaginal Aplasia and Reconstruction," *Best Practice and Research: Clinical Obstetrics and Gynaecology* 24, no. 2 (2010): 185–91. In addition, penis transplant patients have successfully recovered urinary and sexual function. See https://www.reuters.com/article/us-safrica-trans plant/worlds-first-penis-transplant-patient-to-father-a-child-idUSKBN0 OS1HW20150612.

13. For this reason, we believe, with Paul McHugh, that it was an error for physicians at institutions such as Johns Hopkins to attempt to help males born with abnormal genitalia by constructing female "genitalia" and treating these young boys like girls. Such surgeries did not correct a deficiency in physical health and arguably generated significant mental health problems for their subjects. See Paul R. McHugh, "Surgical Sex," *First Things* 147 (2004): 34–38.

14. Obviously sex-change surgeries irreversibly damage the reproductive capacities of patients, but even administering hormones to delay or block puberty can lead to irreversible damage to patients like Jules. Indeed, at present there is no reliable way to suppress pubertal development in males without the risk of rendering the patients permanently sterile.

15. A paradigmatic example of this charge among practitioners of the new medicine is found in Ronit Y. Stahl and Ezekiel J. Emanuel, "Physicians, Not Conscripts: Conscientious Objection in Health Care," *New England Journal of Medicine* 376, no. 14 (2017): 1382. We discuss Stahl and Emanuel at length in chapter 10. For the Obama administration's Health and Human Services mandate asserting that it is unlawful to categorically refuse to participate in gender transition services, see Department of Health and Human Services, "Nondiscrimination in Health Programs and Activities," *Federal Register* 81, no. 96 (2016): 31376–473.

CHAPTER SEVEN   Abortion and Unborn Human Life

1. The American College of Obstetricians and Gynecologists' official policy on abortion says that "induced abortion is an essential component of women's health care." See "Abortion Policy," July 2011, www.acog.org.

2. Ludwig Edelstein, *The Hippocratic Oath: Text, Translation, and Interpretation* (Baltimore, MD: Johns Hopkins University Press, 1943), 3.

3. W. H. S. Jones. *The Doctor's Oath: An Essay in the History of Medicine* (New York: Cambridge University Press, 1924), 23.

4. On human rights and the 1948 Geneva Declaration, see Andreas Frewer, "Human Rights from the Nuremberg Doctors Trial to the Geneva

Declaration: Persons and Institutions in Medical Ethics and History," *Medical Health Care and Philosophy* 13 (2010): 259–68. For a discussion of the changes made in the most recent revision of the declaration, see Ramin Walter Parsa-Parsi, "The Revised Declaration of Geneva: A Modern-Day Physician's Pledge," *Journal of the American Medical Association* 318, no. 20 (2017): 1971–72. For past versions of the declaration, see World Medical Association, "Declaration of Geneva," www.wma.net.

5. The American Medical Association's current position on abortion is terse and noncommittal: "The issue of support of or opposition to abortion is a matter for members of the AMA to decide individually, based on personal values or beliefs. The AMA will take no action which may be construed as an attempt to alter or influence the personal views of individual physicians regarding abortion procedures." American Medical Association, "Abortion H-5.990," last modified 2009, https://policysearch.ama-assn.org.

6. Keith L. Moore, T. V. N. Persaud, and Mark G. Torchia, *The Developing Human: Clinically Oriented Embryology*, 10th ed. (Philadelphia: Elsevier, 2016), 11.

7. For interesting evidence regarding this point, see Helen Pearson, "Your Destiny, from Day One," *Nature* 418, no. 6893 (2002): 14–15.

8. See, in particular, Robert P. George and Christopher Tollefsen, *Embryo: A Defense of Human Life*, 2nd ed. (Princeton, NJ: Witherspoon Institute, 2011).

9. On December 10, 1948, the United Nations ratified the Universal Declaration of Human Rights. See United Nations, "Universal Declaration of Human Rights," www.ohchr.org.

10. See Martin Rhonheimer, *Vital Conflicts in Medical Ethics: A Virtue Approach to Craniotomy and Tubal Pregnancies*, ed. William F. Murphy (Washington, DC: Catholic University of America Press, 2009).

11. Judith Jarvis Thomson, "A Defense of Abortion" *Philosophy & Public Affairs* 1, no. 1 (1971): 47–66.

12. Ibid., 48.

13. Ibid.

14. See Jeffrey Reiman's discussion of the constitutional right to abortion in *Critical Moral Liberalism: Theory and Practice* (Lanham, MD: Rowman and Littlefield, 1996). John Finnis criticizes Reiman's position in "Public Reason, Abortion, and Cloning," *Valparaiso University Law Review* 32 (1998): 361–82.

15. Consider, for example, a mother with no other children, who has a loving husband, strong family support, and a strong devotion to unborn human life; she works, let us suppose, for a pro-life counseling group. Such a mother (but not only such a one) could, we think, reasonably choose in favor

of saving the baby's life. She would be assured the child would be loved and well cared for, and her calling to pro-life witness could lead her reasonably to this choice. But another mother, equally devoted to the unborn but with several other children in need of maternal care, might, in her circumstances, choose in favor of saving her own life. The decision, we stress, is up to her, and she is not without resources for guidance in making that decision. But we think there are limited external grounds on which a third party could criticize one or the other choice.

16. St. Joseph's Hospital and Medical Center, "Bishop Olmsted Announcement: Frequently Asked Questions," accessed May 7, 2018, www .dignityhealth.org.

17. Nicanor Pier Giorgio Austriaco, "Abortion in a Case of Pulmonary Arterial Hypertension," *National Catholic Bioethics Quarterly* 11, no. 3 (2011): 514.

18. For a comparison of the effects on fertility of salpingotomy and salpingectomy, see Femke Mol, Norah M. van Mello, Annika Strandell, Karin Strandell, and Davor Jurkovic, "Salpingotomy versus Salpingectomy in Women with Tubal Pregnancy," *Lancet* 383, no. 9927 (2014): 1483–89, and Xiaolin Cheng, Xiaoyu Tian, Zhen Yan, Mengmeng Jia, Jie Deng, Ying Wang, and Dongmei Fan, "Comparison of the Fertility Outcome of Salpingotomy and Salpingectomy in Women with Tubal Pregnancy: A Systematic Review and Meta-Analysis," *PLoS One* 11, no. 3 (2016): e0152343. For the American College of Obstetricians and Gynecologists' recommendations, see "ACOG Practice Bulletin: Clinical Management Guidelines for Obstetrician-Gynecologists, no. 193," *Obstetrics and Gynecology* 131 (2018): 91–103, www .acog.org.

19. For an argument, which seems sound to us, that the use of methotrexate does *not* necessarily involve intentional killing, see Christopher Kaczor, "The Ethics of Ectopic Pregnancy: A Critical Reconsideration of Salpingotomy and Methotrexate," *Linacre Quarterly: A Journal of the Philosophy and Ethics of Medical Practice* 76 (2009): 265–82.

CHAPTER EIGHT Medicine at the End of Life

1. Leon R. Kass, "Regarding the End of Medicine and the Pursuit of Health," *Public Interest* 4 (1975): 18.

2. World Health Organization, "WHO Definition of Palliative Care," www.who.int.

3. See Timothy E. Quill, Bernard Lo, and Dan W. Brock, "Palliative Options of Last Resort: A Comparison of Voluntarily Stopping Eating and

Drinking, Terminal Sedation, Physician-Assisted Suicide, and Voluntary Active Euthanasia," *Journal of the American Medical Association* 278, no. 23 (1997): 2099–104; Pieter J. J. Sauer and Eduard Verhagen, "The Groningen Protocol—Euthanasia in Severely Ill Newborns," *New England Journal of Medicine* 352, no. 10 (2005): 959–62.

4. National Hospice and Palliative Care Organization, "Preamble to NHPCO Standards of Practice," www.nhpco.org.

5. Atul Gawande, *Being Mortal: Medicine and What Matters in the End* (New York: Metropolitan Books, 2014).

6. A 2006 study found that "on average, patient-designated and next-of-kin surrogates incorrectly predict patients' end-of-life treatment preferences in one third of cases" (David I. Shalowitz, Elizabeth Garrett-Mayer, and David Wendler, "The Accuracy of Surrogate Decision Makers," *Archives of Internal Medicine* 166, no. 5 (2006): 497. In addition, Sharma et al. found that family members are also highly inaccurate in predicting how their loved ones want decisions to be made. See Rashmi K. Sharma, Mark T. Hughes, Mari T. Nolan, Carrie Tudor, Joan Kub, Peter B. Terry, and Daniel P. Sulmasy, "Family Understanding of Seriously Ill Patient Preferences for Family Involvement in Healthcare Decision Making," *Journal of General Internal Medicine* 26, no. 8 (2011): 881–86.

7. The Hippocratic tradition affirmed that the physician should acknowledge and respect the limits of medicine. Consider this statement attributed to Hippocrates in "The Art": "For if a man demand from an art a power over what does not belong to the art, or from nature a power over what does not belong to nature, his ignorance is more allied to madness than to lack of knowledge. For in cases where we may have the mastery through the means afforded by a natural constitution or by an art, there we may be craftsmen, but nowhere else. Whenever therefore a man suffers from an ill which is too strong for the means at the disposal of medicine, he surely must not even expect that it can be overcome by medicine." Hippocrates, "The Art," in *Hippocrates*, vol. 2, trans. W. H. S. Jones (Cambridge, MA: Harvard University Press, 1923), 204–5.

CHAPTER NINE   Last-Resort Options

1. For a discussion of the good of solidarity in this context, see Joseph Boyle, "A Case for Sometimes Tube-Feeding Patients in Persistent Vegetative State," in *Euthanasia Examined: Ethical, Clinical, and Legal Perspectives*, ed. John Keown (Cambridge: Cambridge University Press, 1995), 189–99.

2. See Alan Meisel, Bernard Lo, Timothy E. Quill, and Dan W. Brock, "Last-Resort Options for Palliative Sedation," *Annals of Internal Medicine*

151, no. 6 (2009): 421–24, and, from earlier, Timothy E. Quill, Bernard Lo, and Dan W. Brock, "Palliative Options of Last Resort: A Comparison of Voluntarily Stopping Eating and Drinking, Terminal Sedation, Physician-Assisted Suicide, and Voluntary Active Euthanasia," *Journal of the American Medical Association* 278, no. 23 (1997): 2099–104.

3. See Farr A. Curlin, "Palliative Sedation: Clinical Context and Ethical Questions," *Theoretical Medicine and Bioethics* 39, no. 3 (2018): 197–209.

4. Ira Byock, *Dying Well: Peace and Possibilities at the End of Life* (New York: Riverhead Books, 1998), 193–216.

5. Ibid., 215.

6. For an elaboration of this account of suffering, see Christopher Tollefsen, "Suffering, Enhancement, and Human Goods," *Quaestiones Disputatae* 5 (2015): 104–17.

7. Lord Marchmain's conversion occurs in the final chapter of Evelyn Waugh's *Brideshead Revisited* (New York: Back Bay Books, 1999). The miniseries, directed by Charles Sturridge, was produced by Granada Television and released in 1981.

8. See Curlin, "Palliative Sedation."

9. Arthur Caplan, "Bioethicist Caplan: Brittany Maynard Did Nothing Unethical," *USA Today*, November 4, 2014, www.usatoday.com.

10. See Oregon Public Health Division, "Oregon's Death with Dignity Act—2014," Oregon Health Authority, www.oregon.gov.

11. Brittany Maynard, "My Right to Death with Dignity at 29," CNN, November 2, 2014, www.cnn.com.

12. Oregon Public Health Division, "Oregon's Death with Dignity Act—2014."

13. Ibid.

14. Anthony L. Back, Timothy E. Quill, and Susan D. Block, "Responding to Patients Requesting Physician-Assisted Death: Physician Involvement at the Very End of Life," *Journal of the American Medical Association* 315, no. 3 (2016): 245–46.

15. See www.compassionandchoices.org.

16. Center for Health Statistics and Informatics, "End of Life Option Act," California Department of Public Health, www.cdph.ca.gov.

17. Ian Lovett and Richard Pérez-Peña, "California Governor Signs Assisted Suicide Bill into Law," *New York Times*, October 5, 2015, www.nytimes.com.

18. Robert A. Burt, "The Suppressed Legacy of Nuremberg," *Hastings Center Report* 26, no. 5 (1996): 33.

19. Ibid.

20. The patient's name and some details have been altered to preserve confidentiality.

21. Ludwig Edelstein, *The Hippocratic Oath: Text, Translation, and Interpretation* (Baltimore, MD: Johns Hopkins University Press, 1943, 3.

22. American Medical Association, "Physician Assisted Suicide H-140.952," last modified 2009, https://policysearch.ama-assn.org.

23. Public Health Division, "Oregon Death with Dignity Act, 2017, Data Summary," Oregon Health Authority, February 9, 2018, www.oregon.gov.

24. Disease Control and Health Statistics Division, "Washington State Death with Dignity Act Report," Washington State Department of Health, March 2018, www.doh.wa.gov.

25. Black Americans are significantly less likely to use hospice services. The 2016 "Facts and Figures" published by the National Hospice and Palliative Care Organization and revised in 2018 shows that 8.2 percent of Medicare hospice patients were African American, compared to 86.8 percent who were white. See "Facts and Figures: Hospice Care in America," National Hospice and Palliative Care Organization, revised April 2018, www.nhpco.org . See also Kimberly S. Johnson, Maragatha Kuchibhatla, and James A. Tulsky, "What Explains Racial Differences in the Use of Advance Directives and Attitudes toward Hospice Care?," *Journal of the American Geriatrics Society* 56, no. 10 (2008): 1953–58.

26. Diane Coleman, "Assisted Suicide Laws Create Discriminatory Double Standard for Who Gets Suicide Prevention and Who Gets Suicide Assistance: Not Dead Yet Responds to Autonomy, Inc.," *Disability and Health Journal* 3 no. 1 (2010): 39–50.

27. Richard M. Zaner, *A Critical Examination of Ethics in Health Care and Biomedical Research* (Dordrecht, Netherlands: Springer, 2015), 30–32.

CHAPTER TEN   Conscientious Medicine

1. These arguments lean heavily on a moral distinction and tension between the personal and the professional, whether posed as personal moral values versus professional ethical obligations, personal conscience versus professional conscience, or duties related to personal versus professional integrity. For prominent examples of such arguments, see Julian Savulescu, "Conscientious Objection in Medicine," *British Medical Journal* 332 (2006): 294–97; Julian Savulescu and Udo Schuklenk, "Doctors Have No Right to Refuse Medical Assistance in Dying, Abortion or Contraception," *Bioethics* 31, no. 3 (2017): 162–70; Udo Schuklenk and Ricardo Smalling, "Why Medical Professionals Have No Moral Claim to Conscientious Objection Accommodation

in Liberal Democracies," in *Journal of Medical Ethics* 43, no. 4 (2017): 234–40; Robert F. Card, "Reasonability and Conscientious Objection in Medicine: A Reply to Marsh and an Elaboration of the Reason-Giving Requirement," *Bioethics* 28, no. 6 (2014): 320–26; Eva LaFollette and Hugh LaFollette, "Private Conscience, Public Acts," *Journal of Medical Ethics* 33, no. 5 (2007): 249–54; Howard Brody and Susan S. Night, "The Pharmacist's Personal and Professional Integrity," *American Journal of Bioethics* 7, no. 6 (2007): 16–17.

2. Ronit Y. Stahl and Ezekiel J. Emanuel, "Physicians, Not Conscripts—Conscientious Objection in Health Care," *New England Journal of Medicine* 376, no. 14 (2017): 1380–85.

3. The Professional Obligations and Human Rights policy was issued by the College of Physicians and Surgeons of Ontario, which has state-sanctioned authority over medical practitioners. The college published a fact sheet to explain the policy, www.cpso.on.ca. See *The Christian Medical and Dental Society of Canada v. College of Physicians and Surgeons of Ontario*, 2018 ONSC 579, www.canlii.org.

4. Illinois General Assembly, Public Act 099-0690, SB 1564, July 29, 2016, www.ilga.gov.

5. "Swedish Anti-Abortion Midwife Loses Court Case," BBC, April 13, 2017.

6. Stahl and Emanuel, "Physicians, Not Conscripts," 1382.

7. Ibid., emphasis added.

8. American College of Obstetricians and Gynecologists, "ACOG Committee Opinion No. 385: The Limits of Conscientious Refusal in Reproductive Medicine," *Obstetrics & Gynecology* 110, no. 5 (2007): 1205, emphasis added.

9. Stahl and Emanuel, "Physicians, Not Conscripts," 1383.

10. Eva LaFollette and Hugh LaFollette, "Private Conscience, Public Acts," *Journal of Medical Ethics* 33, no. 5 (2007): 249–54.

11. Howard Brody and Susan S. Night, "The Pharmacist's Personal and Professional Integrity," *American Journal of Bioethics* 7, no. 6 (2007): 16–17.

12. Stahl and Emanuel, "Physicians, Not Conscripts," 1383.

13. American College of Obstetricians and Gynecologists, "ACOG Committee Opinion No. 385," 1205.

14. Dan W. Brock, "Conscientious Refusal by Physicians and Pharmacists: Who Is Obligated to Do What, and Why?," *Theoretical Medicine and Bioethics* 29, no. 3 (2008): 187–200.

15. On page 1205 of the "ACOG Committee Opinion No. 385," they write, "The third criterion for evaluating authentic conscientious refusal is the scientific integrity of the facts supporting the objector's claim. Core to the practice of medicine is a commitment to science and evidence-based practice."

16. Stahl and Emanuel argue that those who refuse patient requests should be treated like conscientious objectors to military service, who "are required to perform alternative service." Stahl and Emanuel, "Physicians, Not Conscripts," 1383.

17. "The military conscientious objector faced real penalties—fines, imprisonment, or alternative service—for resisting conscription." Stahl and Emanuel, "Physicians, Not Conscripts," 1384.

18. Julian Savulescu, "Conscientious Objection in Medicine," *British Medical Journal* 332 (2006): 294.

19. Thomas Aquinas, *Summa Theologiae*, 1-1, q.79, aa12, 13.

20. American College of Obstetricians and Gynecologists, "ACOG Committee Opinion No. 385," 1204.

21. In response to pharmacists who refused to fill prescriptions for emergency contraception, before the FDA made the drug available over the counter, Brody and Night wrote that they "suspect that what the 'conscientious' pharmacist actually objects to, but does not have the nerve to say outright, is the possibility that a woman can engage in sexual activity without having to face the 'moral' consequences of her potentially illicit act." Brody and Night, "Pharmacist's Personal and Professional Integrity," 17.

22. Thomasma defines the conscience of the physician as prudential judgment, adding, "Prudential judgment encompassing medical and value factors in the physician-patient relation is a hallmark of professional conduct." David Thomasma, "Beyond Medical Paternalism and Patient Autonomy: A Model of Physician Conscience for the Physician-Patient Relationship," *Annals of Internal Medicine* 98, no. 2 (1983): 244.

23. Stahl and Emanuel, "Physicians, Not Conscripts," 1380.

24. American College of Obstetricians and Gynecologists, "ACOG Committee Opinion No. 385," 1205, emphasis added.

25. Stahl and Emanuel, "Physicians, Not Conscripts," 1384.

26. Consider this statement in "ACOG Committee Opinion No. 385": "Although respect for conscience is a value, it is only a prima facie value, which means it can and should be overridden in the interest of other moral obligations that outweigh it in a given circumstance" (1207).

27. American College of Obstetricians and Gynecologists, "ACOG Committee Opinion No. 385," 1204.

28. Stahl and Emanuel, "Physicians, Not Conscripts," 1382.

29. Ibid., 1380–81.

30. Ibid, 1383.

31. Ibid.

32. American College of Obstetricians and Gynecologists, "ACOG Committee Opinion No. 385," 1206.

33. Stahl and Emanuel, "Physicians, Not Conscripts," 1383.

34. See John Rawls, *Political Liberalism* (New York: Columbia University Press, 1993).

35. Timothy E. Quill and Howard Brody, "Physician Recommendations and Patient Autonomy: Finding a Balance between Physician Power and Patient Choice," *Annals of Internal Medicine* 125, no. 9 (1996): 765.

36. See Steve Sternberg, "Diagnosis: Burnout," *U.S. News & World Report*, September 8, 2016. See also Tait D. Shanafelt, Omar Hasan, Lotte N. Dyrbye, Christine Sinsky, Daniel Satele, Jeff Sloan, and Colin P. West, "Changes in Burnout and Satisfaction with Work-Life Balance in Physicians and the General US Working Population between 2011 and 2014," *Mayo Clinic Proceedings* 90, no. 12 (2015): 1600–1613.

37. President's Commission for the Study of Ethical Problems in Medicine and Biomedical and Behavioral Research, "Making Health Care Decisions: The Ethical and Legal Implications of Informed Consent in the Patient-Practitioner Relationship," October 1982, 38, https://repository.library .georgetown.edu.

38. Martin Luther King Jr., "A Proper Sense of Priorities" (speech), February 6, 1968, Washington, DC, text available at http://www.aavw.org /special_features/speeches_speech_king04.html.

39. This was said to one of the authors (Curlin) in conversation.

FARR CURLIN is Josiah C. Trent Professor of Medical Humanities at Duke University. He holds appointments in the School of Medicine; the Trent Center for Bioethics, Humanities and History of Medicine; the Divinity School; and the Kenan Institute for Ethics. Curlin has authored more than one hundred and thirty articles and book chapters on medicine and bioethics.

CHRISTOPHER TOLLEFSEN is the College of Arts and Sciences Distinguished Professor of Philosophy at the University of South Carolina. He is the author and editor of numerous books, including *Embryo: A Defense of Human Life and Lying and Christian Ethics.*

Milton Keynes UK
Ingram Content Group UK Ltd.
UKHW030657111224
452151UK00002B/29